YES, YOU CAN!!

Go Beyond Physical Adversity

And

Live Life to Its Fullest

Janis Dietz, Ph.D.

Foreword by Gail Campofiore, M.D.

DEMOS

DEDICATION

*To John, whose love, support, and humor have enabled me
continually to make the choices necessary to say
"Yes, you can."*

*And to my parents, Al and Joan Weinstein, who taught me
to respect values and to get there on my own.*

ACKNOWLEDGMENTS

This book has been eight years in the making - eight years of clipping articles about people who have beaten the odds, people I thought belonged in this book. There are, of course, many more who exemplify the "Yes, You Can Philosophy." To all of them, I extend my thanks for making the choices that are so critical to living your life to the fullest.

One important role model is the late Geri Esten, the founder of the MS Peer Counseling Program. Geri could only move her head for the last 20 years of her life, but she continued to educate herself and to encourage people like me to keep going. Geri, I will always be in your debt.

Drs. Larry Myers and George Ellison, of the UCLA Multiple Sclerosis Center in Westwood, California, have given me support and encouragement during some of my greatest challenges. They helped give this book a purpose.

Zig Ziglar has motivated me for over 20 years. His speeches, tapes, and books have encouraged readers and attendees to strive to be their best. He has lent his considerable talents to the editing of this book and, with a schedule that would tire most politicians, has given me advice that is surely worth more than I could afford to pay for it.

Dr. Gail Campofiore, my personal physician, who wrote the foreword for this book, constantly gives me inspiration with her own struggle with pain and her refusal to give in when she has so many patients who will see only her. Gail is the kind of doctor they just don't make anymore!

CONTENTS

Foreword

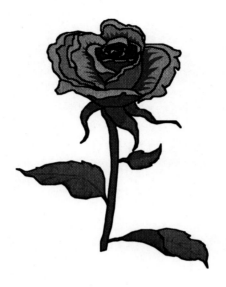

"He who is not busy being born is busy dying."

Bob Dylan

FOREWORD

Gail Campofiore, M.D.

Courage takes many forms, but nowhere is it more evident than in an individual faced with a terminal or debilitating diagnosis who chooses to embrace life and fight for survival. I have had to disclose to many patients the message that their life was going to be drastically different. Sometimes that message was that their life was probably going to end prematurely. Other times, the message was that they have a disease that will slowly ravish their body and strangle their existence.

I am always amazed by the human spirit that says "I won't give in. I will fight and I will lead as productive a life as possible in the time that I have to live." I do not know why some continue to embrace the will to live. For those who give up, life is over and they are waiting to die. For those who choose to fight, life can continue to have many rewards. These are the people who give real meaning to what it is to be happy and productive and these are the people who should be an inspiration to all of us.

As a physician, I am frustrated because I do not know why some choose to live and others choose to wait for death. If I knew the answer, then I would be able to give hope to many more of my patients. My goal is always to help my patient live life to the fullest, no matter how long or short that life is.

Janis Dietz is my patient. She is also my friend and inspiration. I have had major back surgery and I will have to live with pain and reduced mobility for the rest of my life. Life for me is a constant struggle to keep my strength and mobility. Sometimes, when I am feeling sorry for myself and when I question "why me?" I have to remind myself that the physical problems which I face do not compare to those of Janis. How can I complain when she faces life with such a positive attitude. She will not give up whether she walks with a cane or braces or has to use a wheelchair. Multiple Sclerosis may take way some of her physical capacities, but it will not take away her joy of life.

I have dealt with many people who have multiple sclerosis, but never have I seen anyone fight as hard as Janis not to give in. When the disease forces her to make life changes, she doesn't complain; she moves ahead in other directions. When forced to give up her sales job because she no longer could travel, she went back to school and got her doctorate. She is now a university professor teaching youth how to be effective in sales and marketing. Because her disease forced her to change directions, she is having a major impact on the lives of many young people. This would not have happened if Janis has given up. Because she chose to embrace life, she has grown as an individual and has become a role model for both her students and for others struggling to overcome their problems.

This book is a chronicle of her struggle to cope and her success in that effort. It gives proof that life is worthwhile and you can have happiness even if disease or other impairment has taken away some of your capacities. As you read the book, remember that is was not written by academic expert, but was written by someone who has experiences all of the pain and anguish and has made her life fuller and richer in spite of her problems.

Gail Campofiore, M.D. has practiced medicine in Covina, California since 1980. She is board certified in family practice and internal medicine. She holds added certifications in geriatric medicine.

INTRODUCTION

Most of us take normal functions for granted. We have always been able to walk, talk, drink water, read the evening paper, and so forth. When we become unable to handle life or function as we have grown to expect, for whatever reason, we may become angry, confused, and hostile or respond in any number of ways. We may have no experience with a disability, in ourselves or in loved ones. We may have no experience with emotional challenges. We may not see that life itself offers the joy of living as well as the responsibility to live it right. But life should be lived to the fullest extent possible, disability or no disability.

- Everyone is entitled to a full life.
- Even if getting there takes some extra effort.
- Even if getting there takes a long time.
- Even if getting there requires skills you never knew you possessed.
- Even if getting there means you have to work harder than you ever have.
- It is worth it. It has always been worth it.

Life is not a dress rehearsal. We only have one chance to make our dreams come true, to cultivate relationships, and to meet our goals for contributing to life. The recent death of a close relative brought home to me how short a time we are on this earth, and why we should make full use of those few years. There are reminders every day in the news and in the workplace of how short and how precious life can be. If you take some time to think about that, you will appreciate a few minutes of silence more than ever because each minute we live is over in 60 seconds and will never come again.

I wrote this book for you, for all of you; so you need to take it very personally. This book is designed to explore the ways in which anyone can make the most of life. It is designed to celebrate with you your choices as well as mourn with you your losses. You may be reading this book because of depression, because you are having trouble dealing with the loss of a loved one, because you are disabled from an accident or illness, because a divorce has knocked the wind out of your sails, or because of any number of challenges. It is designed to teach, to motivate, and to share.

I have multiple sclerosis. I have had it for twenty-three years and known about it for twelve years. Multiple Sclerosis is often a disabling and chronic disease of the central nervous system, striking adults in the prime of life. Simple everyday tasks can no longer be taken for granted as MS symptoms can run the range from blurred vision to complete paralysis. The course of the disease is unpredictable. Over a period that can run from a few years to decades, many MS patients lose control of their muscles. About a third end up in wheelchairs, but MS is rarely fatal. I define it here as a matter of information only because this book is not about multiple sclerosis—it is about you and me and what we want from our lives. Some of this manuscript is upbeat, and some of it is meant to hit you in the face. All of it is meant to enhance the opportunities you have to live your life to the fullest extent possible. I have found that listing my choices allows for additional options and more control over my life. That is one of the reasons for this book.

You should not read my words with the idea that adapting to your circumstances, whatever they are, is easy. This is hard work, hard work that very seldom ends for most of us. I will be telling you not to "saw sawdust," but instead to have a positive mental attitude, and to never give up. These suggestions do not come lightly. All of it is hard work, but work that will pay off in the end. My message is not that you should concentrate on enjoying what you have left because that is the common sense thing to do. My message is that, even though my suggestions require calling on resources you may not know you have, your life will be better and more satisfying in the long run.

The progressive nature of my particular case has taken me from being an avid runner to someone who cannot walk around the block. When I was diagnosed in 1987, I had been a runner for over fifteen years. I also took aerobic dancing five days a week, rising at 4:45 a.m. to drive to the health club on my way to work in Los Angeles. Before I retired from the Masco Corporation in 1995, my job as a Regional Manager for Peerless Faucet required that I travel over 50% of the time. I managed a $20 million sales territory and 13 sales offices; so much of my time was spent traveling to meet with sales representatives and customers from Texas to Seattle. In the beginning, I told myself that I could handle anything, and that "the worst" would never happen to me. By the end of 1991, I knew I was in trouble because the loss of control in my right foot was endangering my driving ability. This was a big step—to admit to my employer, who owned the car, that I would need modification to continue my duties. Thankfully, the company did not question it. Indeed, the fleet department told me that "your driving record is your driving record," and that the insurance would not be affected. This proved true even when I bought a car myself. One of the things we discover in dealing with life-changing circumstances is that worrying about the modifications we (or our employers) will have to make is sometimes worse than the actual modification. We are fortunate to be living at a time when the ADA requires that employers make accommodations for physical needs, and many times for psychological needs.

Adjusting to limitations forced by illness or injury is very difficult, sometimes the most difficult because of pride. I had to recognize my limitations while, at the same time, refusing to let them interfere with the job I was being paid to do. Although I have worn a brace for over seven years and use a cane frequently, I knew that I had to figure out a way to get the job done in the way that my employer expected and for which I was paid. Problems of balance, fatigue, memory, weakness and cognitive disturbance make living my life in a normal manner a daily challenge. But I do live my life to the fullest and feel very lucky to be able to do so. For me, getting hand controls put on my car was a big step in the direction of freedom, but it did not come without a certain amount of denial. It took a long time to admit that I needed this help, that my illness had progressed to a level where I needed *that* kind of help. When the widow of a good friend first gave me the hand-controls, I told her not to give them to me because I would never need them. She just smiled, and I kept them in my garage until the day came when I had to admit that safety was more important than pride. Had I not availed myself of the aids available, I would not have moved forward in either the corporate world or the academic world.

My choice to enter the academic world was also somewhat serendipitous. A few years after finishing my MBA, I received a call from a former professor, who invited me to apply for a program called the "Forgivable Loan Program," a program designed to recruit women, minorities, and the disabled to teach in California State Schools. The deal was that, if I taught for five years, the State of California would forgive up to $10,000 a year of the cost of a Ph.D. When my mentor called, I said, "Why would I want to get a Ph.D.?" It seemed like much work (which it is), and my travel schedule seemed pretty prohibitive. So I told her that I did not see how I could teach, travel, and go to school at the same time. Then she said, "Why don't you just teach for us?" Apparently my MBA qualified me to teach in college, whereas teaching at lower levels requires an educational certificate.

By now, I was still walking without assistance, but I was starting to realize that the MS was indeed progressing very slowly. I was no longer taking aerobics, but was trying at least walk around in the block in the early morning. So I took my professor up on her offer and taught Sales Management at California Polytechnic University at Pomona. At the end of the semester, I found that it was the most gratifying thing I had ever done. I gravitated to teaching what I had been doing for many years, and the students reacted more positively than I expected. Although I have received many awards and commendations in my 25 years in sales, none of them can compare to a letter from a student who says "You're my hero."

By 1991, I was using a cane to walk all the time and starting to think about changing careers as the disease progressed. I finally decided to apply for that Forgivable Loan from the State of California and apply to graduate school (gulp!). I thought I could go to school at night and continue with my job but not teach while I was going to school. I applied to the Peter F. Drucker Graduate Management Center at the Claremont Graduate School, one of the only part-time Ph.D. programs in the country. The school only accepts ten people a year into their program. I thought I would get the loan but not be accepted into the Claremont program. As it happened, I did not get the loan (I did not mention my disability).

Watch what you wish for because you might get it! One day, in July of 1991, I arrived in Chicago to a message from the director of the Drucker Center, announcing that I was one of two women who had been accepted into the Drucker Executive Management Ph.D. Program. How was I going to pay for this? How was I going to juggle it? Without going into the long process of making the decision, I did decide to go into the program because it seemed to be the best way to move towards attaining the educational credentials I knew were necessary for me to be employable when I could no longer walk. How was I going to pay for it? At the risk of offending you, I will not repeat my husband's words on learning of my acceptance—this program was to cost over $60,000. Although I tend to be a planner and not a spendthrift, I figured I could finance the program with upcoming commissions earned from my sales.

In the beginning of 1992, I got a brace to enable me to walk further, and it added a great deal of freedom to my mobility. That brace, the hand controls, and the love of a wonderful husband have enabled me to be thankful every day for what I have been given, and for the opportunities ahead of me. I finally finished my Ph.D. but not without a great deal of failure along the way. I had to keep the goal in front of me, use the techniques I will discuss in this book, and take advantage of both mechanical and emotional assistance offered along the way.

For other people reading this book, there may be various aids available to help you make the most of your life. Those aids may be hardware, such as a cane, or they may be psychological support, such as a trained professional. You, and only you, have control over your own life. That is why you need to use all the resources available to maximize the way you live *YOUR* life.

Dr. Bernie Siegel, the author of **Love, Medicine & Miracles**, says:

"Live your life now. Don't waste it.
Everybody dies, but there are too many
people who never live."

I have a poster hanging in my office with a picture of a budding daisy. The quote beneath it, from Bob Dylan, is as follows:

"He who's not busy being born is busy dying"

To me, this means that we need to look at our experiences as seeds for growth, *as new opportunities* that hold new challenges. Everyone is entitled to the beauty of a budding flower, the music of Mozart, the hug of a loved one. But not everyone can see the flower, hear the music, or feel the hug. Even so, everyone has the capacity to find beauty and fulfillment in their lives. Our capacity as human beings to adapt to the difficulty of changing circumstances has been the key to our survival on this planet. We are blessed with remarkable abilities to change things, to accept our needs, to improve our lives and to make life easier.

Life, unfortunately, is not fair, but it does offer continuous and considerable opportunities if you work at finding them. It requires work to find that happiness, to find the right way to reach that goal, to find the strength to continue on in the face of physical or emotional hardship. But what worth achieving was ever easy? I used to think you paid a price for success in long hours, hard work and personal sacrifices. Now I realize that you enjoy that process because it is a growth experience that enriches your life. You pay the price for failure--when you decide that life is not worth living to its fullest, that relationships are not worth cultivating, that a job is not worth doing well. You pay a very dear price when you don't take advantage of the opportunities available for you, whatever your physical condition might be. You are alive, and you are a human being! That carries with it a responsibility and joy that animals in other species cannot experience. When someone says to you "How are you?" what do you say? Most people just answer "Fine" without thinking much about it. But if you *do* think about it, you might be able to appreciate what being alive means, and what being "fine" requires.

I have another special perspective on the responsibility we have--that which comes from being an American citizen. Although my ancestors hailed from several parts of the world, I was lucky enough to be born an American. I consider that privilege one that should not be taken for granted--I owe this country all that I have and all that I can contribute because it has given me the joy of a wonderful lifetime. It has also offered me the opportunity to make whatever I wanted out of life. By the way, immigrants to the United States are four times more likely to become millionaires than native-born Americans. They know, from their first feel of American soil, that the opportunities offered here are tremendous. And if they are disabled in any way, they also know that America offers much to anyone, of whatever ability, and in ways that cannot be imagined in other lands.

If you count as home somewhere other than the U.S., be thankful for your homeland's beauty. Since you presumably have made the choice to live where you do, celebrate what it has to offer! It may be special July 4th parades, Thanksgiving gatherings or church potluck dinners. It may be Kwanzaa or All Saints Day. Whatever your current home has for you, it is part of the wonder of living life.

Think about it. And while you are thinking about it, explore with me why life is so precious and how you can adapt its remarkable properties to your own needs, your own goals and your own chosen road to "life, liberty and the pursuit of happiness."

CHAPTER 1

WISHING AND HOPING WON'T CHANGE REALITY

Dale Carnegie, in his best selling book **How to Stop Worrying and Start Living**, used the term "don't saw sawdust" to get across the idea that what's done is done! When we realize this and stop beating the problem into the ground, we can get on with our lives. Have you ever known someone who would not let go of an idea, even when continuing to talk about it was fruitless? I don't waste my time with unproductive complaining and worrying about things that I can't change. Neither did Mark Twain, who said "I can't change the direction of the wind, but I can adjust my sails to always reach my destination." As a matter of fact, studies have shown that athletes who obsess over their mistakes do much worse than athletes who look toward their next opportunity to shine.[1] This example shows you that all human beings catch themselves in situations of distress at certain points of their lives. Whether you are a baseball player who must get over the mistakes made in the last game, or a suddenly disabled salesperson who must find a way to go on with life, the most productive way of dealing with setbacks of any kind is to look toward the future, not back at the past.

Accepting reality is the first, and perhaps the most important, step in living your life to the fullest. After you have accepted reality, you can move on to coping with and to improving on the lemon you have been handed. After you

---

[1] Kushner, H. (1996) **How Good Do We Have to Be**? New York: Little, Brown & Company, p.37.

have accepted reality, you are free to create possibilities for yourself rather than to try to undo what cannot be undone.

Your challenge is real. If it is permanent, such as a physical disability or the death of a loved one, you have to continue to live your life with a revised plan. But you still have to live your life. No one took that responsibility away from you along with the physical loss. So how do you get on with your life if you cannot see, hear, walk or type, drive, etc.? Your ideas, your imagination and your perseverance will answer that question. Retreating from life will not.

Of course, you know many people who can't let go of the past, either because of a wrong done to them, or a good relationship gone wrong. All of us need to get past what is no longer possible, whether it is a contest, marriage, or physical challenge. I must admit to you that the experience of writing this book has made me wake up and realize that I must get past some of my earlier career experiences that still haunt me. It has been very therapeutic. If I use that formula to weigh the pros and cons of reacting to a situation in a negative way, I find it easier to accept what I cannot change. Can I change the fact that I will never be able to run, competitively or otherwise, again? No. So, what do I do about it? I decide that my choices include swimming, and an exercise bicycle, perhaps training with weights. I must focus on what my choices are, not the sawdust of choices that are not to be.

Dick and Mia Holt live in Northern Virginia; they have been married for forty-six years. Dick met Mia when he was stationed in Belgium during World War II. He had spent some time with her family and promised to write; but, before he could, he was wounded at the Battle of the Bulge, rendering him unable to walk or speak clearly for months.

Residual injuries included a two-inch metal plate above his left ear and lifelong comprehension difficulties. To add to their difficulties, Mia was stricken with multiple sclerosis at 53. Along with Dick's back injuries from caring for her, just navigating their home has its challenges. But where others might have given up, the Holts did not. "They accepted their situation, though they were not always dry-eyed, and have made the best of it. They are thankful for the happy moments in a lifetime together that Mia says, somewhat surprisingly, has turned out "just perfect."[2] "What people don't realize is there's so much fun in life," Mia says as she sits propped up in the leather recliner where she spends her days, her legs encased in heavy braces. "I could be sitting here angry about what's happened, but I've learned to adjust. I'm not angry about anything. I've never said 'why me? Why me?' There's no sense in that." When I read her story, I thought how important her attitude is to her mental health and to the Holts' marriage. These people are real life role models.

Dr. Hugh McDonough points out that "It's not what you've lost, but it's what you still have--so use it." In not one of the many conversations I have had with Hugh have I heard him complain about the reality of his disease. He just deals with it.

George and Tena Boehm are "little people" who are 4' and 3'10", respectively. They are very realistic about what they can and cannot do, so they use stools and canes to help

---

[2] Tousignant, M. "A half-century of caring." *The Washington Post,* November 29, 1996.

them get what they want instead of wishing to be taller. They adjust better than most people I've met and are a great inspiration to everyone they meet. Tena recently told me how delighted she is to be taking piano lessons--a few modifications, but she is constantly setting and reaching these kinds of goals. Tena and George have great faith, and they do a lot of public speaking. Their use of reality to improve their lives is an inspiration to anyone. They have been working with a volunteer organization to build houses in depressed areas for several years and have won many accolades for their efforts. When they send us letters from their journeys, all they talk about is what fantastic experiences they are having. Do they have problems because of their height? Most assuredly, but they are not sawing sawdust over it. They are sweeping the floor with their ability and enthusiasm.

Steven McDonald was the sixth member of his family to join the ranks of the New York Police Department—but he was the first to take a bullet in the spine. Ten years later, he still works for the department. "I didn't want to just sit home and do nothing....So we worked it out."[3]McDonald, 36, is on staff as a detective and lectures to students. He faces reality every day; he is also likely to face the sort of criminal who put him in a wheelchair. But Steven uses the reality of his situation to help others, instead of feeling sorry for himself.

Dr. Roger Russell, a psychology professor at the University of La Verne, also faces reality every day. He faces the reality of college students who need his assistance

[3] Vander Pluyn, A. "Real people, real jobs." New Mobility, October, 1996, p.22

to cope with the various aspects of college life and of the myriad conflicts thrown at them during their four-year road to a college degree. But Roger is not any different from any of the other professors on campus. He makes it very clear that his wheelchair, which he uses because of polio, does not hamper his productivity one bit. I can vouch for that because we teach in the same building. I am sure that Roger, like me, wishes he could climb into the stands to watch the football games. But I do not think he wastes much time in those wishes because there are too many other things on which to concentrate; there is too much work to be done!

It dawns on me as I review these words that sometimes I seem too upbeat to be taken seriously. Don't I ever get frustrated or angry? You bet. Several years ago, we went to see a movie with a happy ending about a young woman able to live her life's dreams. Something clicked inside me and the tears flowed such that I could not leave the theater. Today I spent minutes trying to get my foot into my car and yesterday the same amount of time trying to button a blouse. Sure, I get down, just like you and everyone else on this earth, whether they have a disability or not. M y purpose here is not to tell you never to mourn your loss, but to recognize what reality is, and to try to face it in the most productive way possible. The people you admire the most have not ignored their hardships; they have simply chosen to do a "reality check" whenever they are tempted to engage in useless self-pity. As I write these words, last year was the one-year anniversary of the TWA crash of flight 800, which killed over 230 people on the way from New York to Paris in July of 1996. The anniversary services focused on healing and on getting on with life. Those who remain in deep despair are robbing themselves of the opportunities with which they were left.

Dr. David Mohr is the Director of Psychology at the University of California at San Francisco-Mt. Zion Multiple Sclerosis Center. In his research, he has found that people who organize their lives and use their resources wisely are less depressed than others are.[4] They spend their time in productive activities and benefit with a better quality of life.

Mikko Mayeda, an award-winning equestrian, is blind due to multiple sclerosis. Her handicap slowed her down, but it did not stop her. Television viewers throughout the U.S. have seen Mikko display her skillful riding in a dozen difference commercials for the Multiple Sclerosis Society. Mikko says, "If I can do it, you can, too."

Several years ago, the governor of Nebraska came to our attention because he was dating a Hollywood celebrity, Debra Winger. He is good looking, articulate, and carried a political future with him when he left the state house and ran for the Senate. But something else makes Bob Kerry real to us--this Vietnam War hero, who lost a leg in military service, jogs six miles almost daily and has run marathons. He obviously does not deny reality, but he doesn't let it stop him. Bob Kerry must not know how to" saw sawdust" because he is too busy running over it--in politics or on the track!

Beethoven never heard his most important musical achievements. As a matter of fact, when his 5th Symphony was performed, the conductor had to turn Beethoven around so that he could see the audience on their feet applauding his

[4] "Special report: Mood management—the latest word." The Alliance Exchange, February 1999; Biogen, Inc.: Cambridge, MA.

mastery. Losing his hearing did not stop one of the world's greatest musical talents from continuing an incredibly prolific career.

Dr. Merle Bensinger is a psychologist who suffers from Cerebral Palsy. His comments include these words: "Sometimes you have to suffer. The only thing is, you have to have enough experience and knowledge to learn from your suffering rather than become embittered by it. If you get embittered, you're a lost soul." A youth spent living in boxcars and being abandoned taught Merle to adjust and go on rather than rail against his fate and make his life even more miserable.

When I am asked how long I plan to work, I like to remind the questioner that we had a President of the United States in a wheelchair for much of his life. Franklin Delano Roosevelt did not deny reality, but he did not let it stop him because walking was not important in the greater scheme of his contribution to the world. I do, however, find it interesting the lengths he went to conceal the wheelchair, even when it came to statues for public viewing. I can understand it because (I am in no way comparing myself to our last century's greatest president) when I have photos taken for publicity purposes, I prefer the brace and cane to be out of sight. I am not trying to be something I am not, but sometimes the evidence of the disability is irrelevant to the situation. As you go through this book, you will notice that I do not handle the "victim" role very well, and that I lose patience with people whose lives are taken up with talking about their disabilities or other losses. Sawing sawdust. It can poison you.

Paul Hearne has made it his life's mission to improve on reality. Hearne was born with osteogenesis imperfecta, a connective tissue disorder also known as brittle-bone disease. From age four to nine, he lay in a bed in traction and for years after that, he wore a body cast. Fortunately for Paul, his parents encouraged a stream of visitors and diversions for their son. One of those diversions was ham radio, which gave Hearne the education and experience the public school system denied him. In 1971, the dean of Hofstra Law School asked Paul why he wanted to study law. "I want to be a lawyer," Hearne replied.[5] He was told that he would never be able to go to court because of the stairs, or reach books in the library shelves. But Paul Hearne has a habit of getting people to see things his way. Since his graduation from Hofstra Law School in 1974, he has become a forceful voice for the employment and legal rights of people with disabilities.

Neil Jacobson was one of Paul Hearne's Hofstra classmates who told Hearne that one day people would be able to do all kinds of things on laptop computers. Hearne told Jacobson he was crazy. Jacobson, who suffers from cerebral palsy, had the last laugh. He is now in charge of the computer program at Wells Fargo Bank in San Francisco. Neither of these men denies reality. They just keep going until reality meets them halfway.

I am sure you have seen the prayer published by Alcoholics Anonymous: "God grant me the courage to change the things I can change, accept the things I cannot change and the wisdom to know the difference." How true. This prayer,

---

[5] Wolfe, K. (1997). "Crossing disability's borders." *New Mobility*, June, 1997.

used in many forms and by many organizations, very clearly puts into focus how much control you do have over your life and how you can embellish it by separating the sawdust from the worthwhile challenges.

I recently received a letter from an old friend of mine, a marathoner who knows of my past addiction to jogging. He told me he was going to recite the following prayer for me and I want to share it with you:

"Lord Father,
Help me to accept without bitterness this disability which has
suddenly altered my life.
Empower me to see beyond the limitations it imposes.
Teach me how to transform it into a blessing, a means of
deepening my trust in you.
Forgive my moments of frustration, anger, and despondency.
Thank you for the lessons I am learning: the need to treat
everyone with dignity, particularly those who have a
disability: the stroke victim, the blind, the mentally impaired,
the paralyzed, all who are permanently injured.
Lord, I need to discipline myself so that I can achieve
whatever independence is possible for me.
I offer to you the hours of therapy as a silent prayer for all
worn out with sickness and wearied by pain; for all children,
especially those neglected, unloved, abused; and for the
dying. May they find peace with you. For myself, I ask for the
gift of patience, courage and your compassionate love for all
who suffer."

Everyone has his or her own definition of God, but I think this prayer can fit into our need to look outside ourselves for strength. Very few of us get through life alone. We all need to depend on someone or something at various times. For each of us, that someone or something is different at different times in our lives. Part of accepting reality is accepting your responsibility to find outside resources and to use them well.

CHAPTER 2

CONCENTRATE ON WHAT YOU *CAN* DO

That's right, what you *CAN* do. Worrying and spending time complaining about what you *CAN'T* do is unproductive. It just leads to frustration and definitely does not add to the enjoyment of life.

In my own case, losing the ability to jog, which I did for fifteen years, was a devastating blow. Although I never liked other types of exercise, I was able to take up a stationary bicycle and find many positives in it. I am no longer injuring my skeletal structure by pounding my joints against the pavement. By exercising at home, I no longer have to leave the house early, but can get the exercise in the comfort of my own home. I am also able to read business publications while riding my exercise bike, so I am getting the benefit of two activities simultaneously. Now, I'll admit to you that the bicycle does not replace the joy I received from jogging, but I have chosen to use the choice I do have, that of utilizing other methods of exercise open to me, rather than to mourn over the choices I no longer have. Perhaps you are getting the hang of my strategy.

I also found that I could contribute to the MS Society by serving as a public speaker and counseling newly diagnosed MS patients, as well as helping with the fund raising activities. I have found these activities to be very gratifying and worthwhile. Believe me, there are many ways that you can add to the good of society by using skills that you possess.

You may be familiar with another example of concentrating on remaining abilities--the Academy Award winning film "My Left Foot", which chronicled the life of Christy Brown, an Irishman with cerebral palsy who taught himself to paint with his left foot. In the movie, which includes an exhibition of his paintings, Christy says, "I have made myself understood to people in all parts of the world and that's something we would all like to be able to do." Right on, Christy!

One of the members of the President's Council on Mental Retardation is a young woman with Down's syndrome. She has been pictured on television wearing her motivational button, with "Downs" crossed out and "UP" put in its place. She is most certainly concentrating on the talents that she has, and making the most of them.

Several years ago, we took a wonderful cruise to Alaska and met many people using canes and wheelchairs. They did not let their challenge stop them because they realized that they could still enjoy the majestic scenery of our 49th State. In everyday life, I meet many people with the same physical problems as many of my fellow passengers. The difference is that some of them let their problems stop them. With the many accommodations now available to people with disabilities, there are many more things we all can do!

Dianne Pilgram is the director of the Cooper-Hewitt, National Design Museum, a New York branch of the Smithsonian Institution. She is an art and design historian. She is also in a wheelchair. Diagnosed with multiple sclerosis in 1978, she never stopped working. She loved working at the Cooper-Hewitt, where she has a public platform from which she can talk about the Americans with Disability Act and from which she can explore solutions with the creativity for which her education has prepared her. Dianne says that she is not different from what she was before she needed a wheelchair, except that she has grown stronger psychologically. She can most definitely contribute more to society from this vantage point than if she set her goals lower because of her disability.[6]

Since I have had the benefit of a brace to counter the lack of control I have in my foot, I have been wearing Easy Spirit casual shoes, even for work, because that is the only shoe that will fit over the brace. When I was buying some Easy Spirit shoes in a variety of colors at Nordstrom some months ago, I remarked to the salesman, who had been so helpful in fitting me, that I had given away several thousand dollars worth of pumps and heels that I could no longer wear. He picked me up out of my sorrow when he remarked: "you're lucky you can walk!" Of course, he was right. That was just the remark I needed. I needed to appreciate what I could do and to stop dwelling on what I could not do.

Merle Bensinger, the Sacramento psychologist, used his superb memory, and lessons learned from years as an orphan, to overcome his cerebral palsy. The Los Angeles Times quotes Bensinger: "If you're alive and growing inside, you attract people to you. You can't do that unless you have something to give."

"Find something you are passionate about." Those are the words of Tom Peters, a noted management consultant

---

[6] Pilgrim, D. (1997). "Historic buildings can be people-friendly." *Messages*, sponsored by Berlex Laboratores, May, 1997. Vol 3, No.2

and author. Looking around at the choices for activities, surely you can find something in which to get involved. As Dale Carnegie's teachings remind us, we can only think of one thing at a time. If you are concentrating on which of your talents to cultivate, you won't have time to feel sorry for yourself. But remember that you *can* matter and that you *do* matter--all the time!

The husband of a friend lost his leg to a mysterious infection last year. His friends marvel at his positive attitude. I was interested in a conversation with him recently to hear him say "I will not give in to 'it.'" In other words, the leg is only part of what he is. He has returned to golf, which he never thought he would be able to do and has found that he was able to continue many of the things he likes to do. I have never heard him talk about all the things he cannot do.

I have the pleasure of serving on the Board of Trustees for the Southern California Chapter of the National Multiple Sclerosis Society. It is part of what I *can* do. One of our members, who is very active in the entertainment industry, has suffered for twenty-eight years from numbness caused by multiple sclerosis. In a recent newsletter, he wrote that the activity he missed most was tennis, where he had lettered in high school and college. But then he watched actor Christopher Reeve, paralyzed from the neck down by a riding accident, courageously say, "You have to be grateful to be alive, and you have to take risks."[7] The next day, without telling anyone, he went out and purchased a tennis racquet. His comment about his first lesson was "The timing was a

---

[7] "Action News," National Multiple Sclerosis Society, Southern California Branch, December, 1996

little off, but I was hitting a tennis ball again." The partner with whom he plays and who also has MS, commented " it's not exactly tennis the way I used to play, but instead of worrying about that, I look at the bigger picture and feel it is a joy to be able to do something I love to do but thought I could never do again." What did these people do? They concentrated on what they *could* do, which was to play a slightly modified game of tennis.

I recently took a lesson from my colleague on the MS Board—I went out and bought an exercise video! I took aerobics for about ten years, and miss it dearly. I used to like the Richard Simmons (® Hometime Videos) tapes because they were so upbeat, but when I lost much of the use of my right leg and my right arm, it seemed foolish to attempt the exercises that I used to do in aerobics. After I read my friend's article about his return to tennis, I went down to a video store and purchased the tape. I then waited. I waited for my husband to go out of town. If I was going to attempt this, I did not want to risk his laughter as well as the $20 cost of the video! On a recent three-day weekend, I put the tape on and, with my one good leg and one good arm, had a blast! Did I do everything on the video that Richard Simmons did? No, but I bet a lot of the home audience doesn't, either! I did what I *could* do, which was more than I expected!

Speaking of Christopher Reeve, you may be aware of the attention the media has paid his comeback to directing and acting. I can think of no better example of concentrating on remaining abilities. His wife said in a recent newscast, "We can't let *it* be bigger than us."

Greg Smith is a member of two minority groups—America's largest, those people who are handicapped (50 million), and America's second largest minority group, African Americans. Greg and his partner, Todd Himball, co-produce a radio show called *On a Roll* in Phoenix, Arizona. It is the only syndicated radio talk program for the disabled community. Greg was bitten by the broadcast bug back in junior high school. To quote Greg, "The other kids were out riding their bikes and running around. I couldn't do that; so I found things I could do.[8]" He could keep score and he could do play-by-plays. In high school, he became "the voice of the Mustangs" at South High in Downers Grove, Illinois. His dad used to carry him up the stairs to the press box and then back down the stairs at half-time to play in the marching band. "I knew then that radio was something I wanted to do," said Greg. "It had the deep voice, and it didn't require physical strength." Along the way, Greg earned a degree in broadcasting from the Walter Cronkite School of Journalism at Arizona State University. He wanted to be a sales representative for a talk station in Phoenix, but because he was in a wheelchair due to muscular dystrophy, the station did not think he had the energy level to do it. So he did research; eventually, he bought time on KFNN in Phoenix, where he launched "On a Roll." Although Greg's example is one that shows a very long period of persistence and rejection, it is perfect for this chapter because Greg is concentrating on the doors that are open to him, not on those that are closed.

Many disabled people must change professions or quit work completely. Although I chose to pursue my Ph.D. in part because of the need to find a job not as physically demanding as my sales career, the opportunity to use my

---

[8] Maddox, S. (1997). "Greg Smith: he's on a roll." *New Mobility*, April, 1997

motivational skills and sales experience has benefited me tremendously. This opportunity would not have occurred had I chosen to continue with the profession I had known for seventeen years.

An optometrist I know has had to change his activities due to his disability, but he gives everyday with his leadership of the local MS support group. He said to me simply, "Don't give up." He tries to keep active, to give people something to which to look forward. I have many examples of people who have founded and supported these groups because they have the time and the desire to contribute in this way.

Tom Carr, another MS patient who has changed his activities in recent years, spent a long time telling me about the book he and his wife wrote, about his religious devotion and his change from Nuclear Engineering to Public Relations at Bechtel. It was obvious during our conversation that Tom is delighted with his life and feels it is in good balance. He told me that "People have to do whatever they can do." I don't know about you, but that surely motivated me!

Robert Metcalf is a CPA with many tax clients, practicing law and selling securities on the side. He is also a quadriplegic. After several years of practicing accounting, he decided that "I've got to be better than the average accountant.[9]" So he went to night school to earn a law degree. One of the comments I found most interesting was "Whether it's a disability or anything else that hinders you in the

---

[9] Petzinger, T. "Accountant Metcalf knows firsthand give and take of takes." *The Wall Street Journal*, August 11, 1995,P.B1

business or professional world, you've got to be head and shoulders above the average."

What you *can* do is not always the art of producing or making something. My nephew, David, has Down's syndrome. He lives in State College, Pennsylvania. Although my sister was afraid of "the unknown" when he was born, she and the other members of their family have found that David adds great joy to their family unit. David shares easily, smiles with delight and truly lends an extra dimension to all his relationships. He may not be able to say his ABCs as fast as his sister and brother did at his age, but his every accomplishment is a delight to his parents. In a speech to an advocacy group on mainstreaming these special children into the educational system, my sister told them that "He has something nobody else has. It is that something extra that you will feel if you are lucky enough to get to know my son David." My sister and her husband, as well as their other two children, spend their time concentrating on what he *can* do.

Some thoughts on what you *CAN* do:

1. Everyone is good at something and not so good at something else. What does the disability do for you? Offer a new career that is not as stressful, a new surrounding, a chance to go back to school and learn a new skill? When you start to explore your options with an open mind, you will be surprised at how many alternatives there are that you may have never considered.

2. Things happen. Opportunities come up, people you run into need just the skill you have or there is an opening

somewhere that just occurred. I don't know whether to call it fate, but somehow the right thing will come along. Just don't give up.

3. If you can't walk, a wheelchair or an Amigo will give you your mobility back and freedom to continue your life. The late Geri Esten, the founder of the Los Angeles Peer Counseling Service for the Multiple Sclerosis Society, said, "You have to figure out what you want and find a way to do it." Geri could move only her head, yet lived a full life as a licensed Marriage and Family Counselor. She concentrated on the remarkable listening and communication skills she had. It did not take too long to stop noticing that she could not move her arms and legs, because Geri concentrated on what she *COULD* do. She once took a trip to Washington, D.C.--she never gave a thought about whether or not she *COULD* do it! By the way, she reported having a wonderful time.

4. Here are some other remarkable people:

* Skye Osborn, a Nevada writer, wanted to go on a climbing expedition in Colorado. Her multiple sclerosis forced her to use a cane, and she wore off the tip of the cane in the process of the hike. But she made it and stood high overlooking the Colorado Mountains in triumph.

*Candace Cable-Brooks is one of the premier women wheelchair athletes in this country. She cannot walk, but she uses her arms to outdistance her competitors in races and sets an example for anyone with this kind of challenge.

*I know of a young orthopedic surgeon in Los Angeles who is one of the most respected members of the medical staff. Her polio and thus, the need to use two crutches do not stop her from using her knowledge and skill to do exactly what she wants to do.

* You may have seen Stephen Hawking interviewed on television or in reviews of his best selling book, <u>A Brief History of Time</u>. Dr. Hawking is purported to be the greatest mind since Einstein. Due to amyotrophic lateral sclerosis (Lou Gehrig's disease), he can only move his thumb. He communicates with a computer. Dr. Hawking is a full-time professor at Cambridge University. He even has his own fan club! He concentrates on what he CAN do, which is to develop and teach the ideas his brilliant mind conceives. Is not the scientific world lucky that Stephen Hawking disregards his disability and looks instead at how he can best contribute to the world.

*Dr. Hugh McDonough recently received his PhD from the University of Southern California. His thesis, painstakingly typed with three fingers on his home computer, was on "Attitudes Toward People With Disabilities in America." He had to leave State employment in 1983, but went on the get his master's degree from USC and to teach part-time at California Polytechnic University, where he has applied for a full-time job. He is also working to establish a disability administration program at USC to teach people who are not disabled how to employ people who are. I imagine that Hugh will look back on this change in his career with satisfaction because of the impact he can have on other disabled people.

No one does everything well. The most brilliant concert pianist may not be able to balance his or her checkbook! Even able-bodied people have to make choices based on what they do particularly well and to eschew those that may lead to failure. By concentrating on what you can do, you are only following the natural selection of skills a little further.

I have received motivation from the writings and lectures of Zig Ziglar for almost 20 years. In his book <u>Top Performance</u>, Zig mentions his sister-in-law, who has multiple sclerosis. He expected that, when she visited, she would not be able to navigate the stairs in their new home. She told him that she could do anything she wanted, as long as she did it "one step at a time." I find that attitude helpful because many people are surprised that I continue to travel with the limitations my legs have placed on me. No problem; I just take into consideration how much longer it will take me to get between gates and make arrangements for chairs and places to rest. By the way, I, too, live in a two-story house that was purchased before my MS started to progress. I handle it one step at a time, just like Zig Ziglar's sister-in-law. Taking challenges one-step at a time, whether they are physical or mental, simply makes more sense.

CHAPTER 3

EXPLORE WHAT POSITIVES HAVE COME OUT OF THIS EXPERIENCE

You know the old story about the cloud with the silver lining. I really believe that you can find good in most situations, though you may have to look extra hard for it.

Maybe it is a new career that you would not have attempted had it not been for the disability. A teaching career had not occurred to me until I faced the need to do something that did not require walking. But I have found that teaching is the most gratifying activity I have ever undertaken, and I am thankful for the chance to discover this alternate career--indeed, a career that may make me happier than the one I have spent most of my adult life pursuing. If I compare a $1 million order for Peerless faucets from Home Depot to a letter from a student telling me "You taught me so much," it is no contest! My goal in life has been to make a contribution. Although I know that I made many fine contributions in my seventeen years in the home center industry, the chance to make the kind of contribution that enriches a college student's life is far more gratifying.

Wilma Rudolph, as a child, walked with the aid of a leg brace, but ran to three Olympic gold medals and inspired a generation of future champions. She was an example of the good that can come out of relentlessly pursuing a goal. One of her disciples, Benita Fitzgerald, "said that she placed a poster of Rudolph over the bed in her dormitory room while attending the University of Tennessee. Fitzgerald later won the gold medal in the 100-meter hurdles at the 1984 Summer Olympics in Los Angeles."[10]

I mentioned that I have replaced my morning jog with a stationary exercise bicycle. While I was pursuing my Ph.D., I was able to use the reading rack in the bike to get some of the reading done--I most certainly consider this a positive that has come out of my change in routine.

Earlier, I mentioned Tom Carr, the Bechtel Engineer. Tom told me that he had the opportunity to play professional tennis but chose to stay in school and finish his engineering degree. Looking back on his disability, which struck shortly after he finished college, Tom is very thankful that he made the choice he did.

A few years ago, I heard a friend, who lost her husband and overcame breast cancer in the same year; say "When one door closes, another one opens." I have heard this statement many times, but it really hit home when she said it. Here is a woman who has much to feel sorry about. But she does not. She just keeps opening those doors! Recent downsizing in the aerospace industry forced her into early retirement, but she is now exploring the positives of extra time to spend with her grandchildren.

Another woman I met on a recent plane ride has had cancer for eighteen years. She has her own counseling service and has thrown herself into working in Europe to create more cooperation among businesses. She seems glad that she thought her time was limited because she has accomplished

---

[10] Harvey, R. "Olympic legend Wilma Rudolph dies." *The Los Angeles Times*, November 13, 1994.

so much. Indeed, her time does not seem to be limited now-I wonder if that is a coincidence?

I am sure you know recovering alcoholics who lecture to other groups. Their problem enables them to affect other people in a positive and stimulating way. The positive aspects of the help that comes out of these experiences are a very real contribution to the lives of others.

In recent years, a number of celebrities have come forth to publicize their struggle with cancer. By sharing their experience with the public, they have prompted many people to seek care in ways that promote early detection.

Another celebrity whose struggle has inspired us is Patricia Neal, whose Broadway and Hollywood stardom came crashing down when she suffered a series of three massive strokes that left her in a coma for weeks. She fought her way back. Today she acts, lectures around the world, and devotes much of her time to the Patricia Neal Rehabilitation Center in Knoxville, Tennessee.

Ed Turner says that misfortune can be a gift, that the misfortune of his injury in a diving accident and the resulting physical condition made him a better man. He has found strength and perseverance that he never knew he had. His faith in God has grown. He also says that he has had more success in life since his injury, which broke his neck, than before. He has been able to build a pizza restaurant from a small place into three full-service restaurants employing over one hundred people. Ed says that those who have encountered misfortune must make their way back into life, for if they do not, they cannot go forward, and they themselves will "wither in bitterness."[11]

I know a lady who volunteers daily at a hospital near my home. Her polio keeps her in a wheelchair, but I know she gets a great deal of pleasure from helping people in this way. The example she sets, and the special care she gives, are positive impacts on other people's lives that would not have occurred if she were not there.

The fast track is a sign of our times. But sometimes we do not catch our breath long enough to weigh the value to us of the activities we choose. Is it better to work part-time for a non-profit organization or run from plane to plane? Which meets your life's goals? Your goals will certainly change with time, but you should always update what you really want out of live within the context of your situation. Remember that your goals would have changed with time even if you were not challenged with a disability.

When a disability strikes someone during his or her prime earning years, as it has me, the value of money has to take on a different perspective. I think I am happier now that my career priorities have changed.

At the beginning of this book, I said that we all take normal functions (in my case, walking) for granted. Often it is only when we lose these functions that we realize how precious they are. One of the books I highly recommend is **Head First**, by the late Norman Cousins. Norman Cousins was the Editor of "The Saturday Review" for over twenty-five years before he accepted an appointment to the faculty

---

[11] "Quickie Listens" *Quickie Chronicles*, Winter, 1997.

at UCLA. He sought to find proof that positive attitudes are not merely moods, but biochemical realities. He pointed out that "Life is the ultimate prize, and it takes on ultimate value when suddenly we discover how tentative and fragile it can be. The essential art of living is to recognize and savor its preciousness..." Amen to that!

Perhaps the most positive benefit of my illness is that I do not take movement for granted any more. I appreciate every day that I can walk. I find that I do not let little things bother me any more, and I have been able to modify my Type A behavior in a positive manner (translation: Type A people push the elevator button several times). When I recently got into a squabble with a co-worker about abuse of power, I put it into perspective and let the situation go.

I am more relaxed about my life. I am sorry I waited this long to smell those roses! The positives that come out of a disabling accident or illness will be there, but they will not be immediate; in many cases, they will not be obvious. But they WILL be there!

For you old married ladies out there, you know that no marriage partner is perfect. Men seem to have problems finding the clothes hamper and they have problems concentrating on more than one thing at a time—do not ask them to choose between the television set and talking to you unless you are prepared for the outcome! But we wives, I am sure, are the subject of jokes when the guys "bond" about our propensity to change the subject without warning, to use the grocery store as a bank, or to always want them to take us places where they have to wear a tie. If you are lucky, as I am, you have a spouse who helps you through the tough times without smothering you. Will I tell you that a positive of my illness is a great marriage? No, but I think I appreciate that great marriage, and make sure not to take it for granted. It is the most precious thing I have.

CHAPTER 4

COUNT YOUR BLESSINGS

I consider myself luckier than most because I have had a wonderful life, with a wonderful family and the chance to get an education. Not everyone is as lucky as I am, but most people can look at people less fortunate than they are-- people in other countries, other circumstances, people without resources, who are in situations far worse than their neighbors. I am not saying that it is not frustrating to watch other people run, take aerobics, even walk around the park. Those were activities that were very important to me. As a matter of fact, I was addicted to jogging in the same way that some people are addicted to alcohol. Not being able to walk around the block is as frustrating to me as it is to anyone else who loves to jog, but I have to remind myself constantly of how lucky I am to have had fifteen years of running and to live such a high-quality life. Crying over the loss of my ability to run is not a productive activity. I like to concentrate on ways to improve the quality of my life, not drag it down by mourning something about which I *do not* have a choice.

You may be familiar with Richard Dreyfuss, the popular actor. His wife, Jeremy, has Lupus. Lupus is a disease characterized by tumors, weakness and many hospital stays. In a television interview, she chronicled how she spends her energies trying to draw attention to Lupus, but she also said something very important: "The only thing I know is that I'm so happy to be here that I'm not going to let anything get in the way of living my life!"

I recently had a conversation with a lovely lady who has lived almost her entire sixty-seven years with polio. She told me that she never knew what it was like to run, jump and live a normal life. But she raised three children with her limited ability to walk or stand. Can you imagine raising babies with that kind of handicap? Betty told me that they used to come to her to be spanked! We agreed on one very important issue about accepting life's problems--we both have terrific parents thus we thank them for our childhood! Betty's mother told her, "You don't need legs to be a person." Her daughter told her that if she could have any wish, she would want to pass on the kind of childhood that Betty had given her children. Betty took that strong parental encouragement and has proceeded to live her life to the fullest, volunteering in several community centers. Betty has counted her blessings her entire life. There are many, many people who are better off because of Betty's attitude.

There are five senses--sight, hearing, touch, taste and smell. If you have even one of these, you can count your blessings. Helen Keller certainly did and became an example of remarkable contribution to humanity. Try this: take some time tomorrow to concentrate on what it would be like to lose even one sense—for instance, the ability to smell the air and the flowers, or even the smog). By the end of the day, you will have a greater appreciation for that sense. Then the next day, try another sense where you can again count the blessings of having that sense intact. If we all did this exercise monthly, we might find a new delight in the wonders of nature.

Delight in small things!!!

I am one of the 50% of Americans who are first or second generation Americans--not a day goes by that I do not feel extremely thankful for this good luck! As Americans, we enjoy the greatest medical treatment in the world, the best facilities for the handicapped (if you don't believe me, try traveling to Europe in a wheelchair), and the most transportation alternatives. Living in the United States is a blessing all by itself, and needs to be cherished.

My husband says that I am easily entertained and delighted. This is one of his many ways of teasing me, but it is okay with me. I take real joy in, among other things:

--sharpened pencils

--my first cup of coffee on an early morning flight

--Daffodils

--Christmas music

--the American Flag and the National Anthem

--watching small children

--the sight of my husband's car in the driveway

--a compliment

--the completed laundry on Saturday

--paper clips

And I have learned NOT to get so upset about the following:

--delayed flights

--the Los Angeles traffic

--rude waiters

--fallen soufflés

--lost arguments

What is my point? My point is that one should, as the younger generation has been known to say, "Chill out", and, as a small frame in my living room points out, "Smell the roses." You are special. You *can* do many things that other people do not have the opportunity or ability to do. There are no two people like you in the world!

Several years ago, I read a book entitled **I Raise My Eyes to Say Yes**, about the life of Ruth Sienkiewicz-Meyer, a forty year-old victim of cerebral palsy. She communicates with the collaborating author by guiding her eyes toward the words she wants him to use in the story. Ruth recounts an experience at a rehabilitation center in New Hampshire where they played a game very similar to musical chairs, except played with wheelchairs and crutches. I believe that Ruth took as much delight in that game and in being with her friends as you and I did when we played it on our feet.

Puff out that chest and make your own list of things to delight in the fact that you can do- some of them may be the following:

--you have 10 fingers

--you can yodel (I can't)

--you are ambidextrous (I wish I were)

--you have a photographic memory!

--you have lots of friends

Being on this earth and waking up every day, in whatever condition, is a lot to be thankful for--and I should be thankful a lot more often than the fourth Thursday in November! Because I grew up on the East Coast, in Alexandria, Virginia, and lived in Rhode Island for seven years, I can claim plenty of experience with snow. I have lived in Los Angeles for more than twenty-two years now, but I have never taken for granted the weather here. I never take for granted the fact that I do not have to trudge over a snow-covered campus to get to my classes. I am somewhat frustrated when my students complain that "it is cold outside (45°)." They do not want to hear about the miles I walked to school in the snow-well, _ mile anyway—so I don't launch into a tutorial on counting your blessings. But they will learn, and I hope they will realize someday how good they have it. Personally, I like snow when it is on the other side of a pane of glass.

The next time you are caught in traffic, look at the person in the car next to you and try to figure out what kind of life he or she lives. Chances are, you would not trade places with him or her. Or look at the architecture on the buildings. Or just relax and turn the radio to something soothing. You can produce your own stress relief with just some soothing music and a few thoughts of your blessings.

Yes, take delight in some of life's little pleasures.

There are many.

CHAPTER 5

PASS IT ON: HOW CAN YOU HELP OTHERSOVERCOME THEIR PROBLEMS THROUGH YOUR EXPERIENCE?

You can be a great motivator and an example for other people trying to come to terms with a disability.

When I first joined the MS Speakers Bureau, I thought I would use my public speaking skills to pass on my knowledge to other people. But I met a lady there whose smile I have never forgotten. Her name is Edna Marie Smith and her face radiates with good cheer! She says, "There are two sides to everything--good and bad--even multiple sclerosis. If you smile a lot and laugh a lot, you will attract people." I still laugh at one of Edna's comments: "You can still be the life of the party; you just can't monopolize the dance floor!" Edna helped me at a difficult time in my life and I can only hope that I can do the same for someone else some day.

Being able to talk with someone else in the same situation is very helpful and important for anyone with a disability. I found that being a peer counselor for the MS Society allowed me to use my motivational skills in a helpful manner. My objective is to help other people overcome their fear or the anger they may feel because of their disability. My experiences and those of others can be a big help in breaking down some of these feelings.

Stephen Hawking, the noted British physicist I mentioned earlier, has made many contributions to causes for the disabled and learning-impaired, using the strength of his notoriety and helping advance those causes in very important ways.

Syndicated columnist Dianne Piastro has had to make many lifestyle changes as her limitations have progressed. But her career change has put her more in touch with people she can help. "I've found a career I can do at home that helps me and, I hope, that helps others as well." Dianne is using her energies to reach out to other people and thus she gets more in return.

The late Bill McGowan was Chairman of MCI. A hard charging businessman his entire life, he had difficulty in slowing down when he underwent a heart transplant. But Bill McGowan became deeply involved in promoting transplants, so much so that he pledged $1 million to the University of Pittsburgh Medical Center for clinical study of an implantable heart-assist device that could obviate the need for donor hearts. Not only did Bill McGowan cut his workweek to the 40-hour variety most of the time, but he used his time to help others improve their chances.

Most people do not see much humor in being disabled. John Callahan, who draws cartoons for the "Willamette Week" in Portland, Oregon, has developed quite a following due to his humor in his cartoons. "His work speaks to amputees, recovering alcoholics and people dealing with all manner of tragedy and pain.[12]" Because his work contemplates the ridiculous situation in which disabled people find themselves, John is making a contribution to

---

[12] *Los Angeles Times*, July 28, 1991

people who, more than most, need to see humor in their lives.

From 1982 to 1986, Bob Wieland, a disabled Viet Nam veteran, "walked" across America using his arms, raising money for the homeless. He raised $350,000 in his three years, eight month and six day travail. He helped many people at the expense of great effort, but he did use what he had to help them in ways that exhaust most of us to even contemplate! But wait, then he did it again! In 1996, Weiland cycled across America using his hands with the goal this time to raise money for children. A champion weightlifter, marathon runner and tri-athlete, "he hopes that through his physical accomplishments he can inspire junior and senior high school students to elevate their own individual standards."[13]

Helen Keller remains a hero to all of us. Her courage and accomplishments, amid a devastating loss of abilities, inspire us to cope with our own physical challenges. I recently saw a television show outlining some parts of her life. One quote that I feel belongs in this chapter was "dark as my part may seem to them, I have within me a majestic light." I think Helen Keller helped and, through her work, continues to help many people overcome handicaps to reach just a little harder for what they know is out there for them.

I am not sure if it was an advertisement or human interest story, but I read a section of the Los Angeles Sunday Times that described how Marilyn Hamilton, a Fresno businesswoman who had become paralyzed after a hang-

---

[13] Duncan, M. "Inspiring trip across America." *The Daily Bulletin*, December 6, 1995.

gliding accident, enlisted the help of friends with backgrounds in aerospace engineering to design a fast, light-weight wheelchair. Marilyn obviously was not content to struggle with the standard sixty-five plus pound wheelchair. She found a way to help herself and others in the process. The pictures show colors, a chair draped in the American Flag and parts made of lightweight metals that enable them to glide almost effortlessly. I frequently see people with this kind of chairs at airports and marvel at the innovation. I am sure many people other than Marilyn Hamilton have been involved in inventing equipment to make one's life easier, but it is an example of someone who used her experience to help others live a better life.

Another example of technology being created out of necessity is the proliferation of mechanical typing and speaking aids for the disabled. Examples include the following:

•Computer software that understands voice commands, so that fingers are not necessary ($59 from IBM)

•Computerized "sip and puff" machines, which can switch on the TV, telephone a friend and play computer games with a light puff into a plastic straw

•Wheelchairs that stand up, making it possible for the disabled to greet someone face-to-face, to take a book from a shelf or to dance with their loved one

About twenty years ago, I remember seeing a television program focusing on Max Cleveland, the head of the Veterans Administration at the time. As I watched this man without arms and legs play basketball (using the stumps of his arms), I said to myself, "I'll never complain about anything again." I wish I could say I've lived up to that promise, but I vividly remember the episode and have repeated the story many times to other people having a rough time with a physical problem. Max Cleveland took his experiences and helped others like himself to make the most of their lives. His example has, I am sure, helped thousands and thousands of people to make the best of what they have left. I can't think of a more appropriate person to head an organization dedicated to our Veterans. In November of 1996, he was elected to the Senate from the State of Georgia—how is that for making full use of non-physical faculties!

There are many books published which give examples of ways to enrich one's life. I do not know about you, but my memory is not good enough to remember everything I have read during my 25 years in sales. So I read them again. I have read Zig Ziglar's **See You at the Top** and Dale Carnegie's **How to Stop Worrying and Start Living** many times. You can use your experiences and special skills to motivate, to listen, to "be there" and to communicate in just the right way.

As a college professor, it pains me to see the trauma that many of my students go through as a natural consequence of growing up. I would love to spare them the pain of their first failed romance, their first bad grade, their first loss of an election. But I cannot. All I can do is be there for them and assure them that my failures would make theirs look like a bump on the knee. That is how I use my experiences to try to help them. Of course, I choose the failures I share with them carefully (as you can well imagine), but I need to use my human experiences to help them accept their challenges.

Several years ago, Ken Blanchard (**One Minute Manager**) and Don Shula (Miami Dolphins) wrote a book entitled **Everyone's a Coach**. It is a very good book for parents, teachers, coaches, and for anyone who has to coach *himself or herself.* And *you* have to coach yourself. You are most qualified for the job, you have the most to gain, and you are holding the stopwatch. You have to set goals for yourself, get yourself back up when things do not go well, and make decisions about your future. In that way, your experiences can help you along with others. Do not overlook your role as your own coach. The people I mention in this book have had to coach themselves through many challenges. The way they did it, and do it, was to be their own cheering section, to tell themselves they could do it, even if no one else thought they could. That kind of victory is even sweeter. Coach yourself every day, be nice to yourself, and share the benefits of your own coaching with others.

I am sure you know how therapeutic it can be to have someone with whom to share your "challenges". Either they have been there, or you have; and you have the benefit of real life experience to talk about. If by listening or sharing your experience, you can enrich someone else's life at a time when he or she so desperately needs help, you can take pleasure in knowing that you have made a very important difference to that one person. Who among us would eschew that kind of opportunity? Because the challenges I am addressing in this book cover many challenges, including emotional challenges, the loss of a loved one, and physical challenges, the opportunity to share experiences with others as a way toward healing becomes one of the most important ways we cope.

CHAPTER 6

WHEN OTHERS WANT TO HELP

Several years ago, I was sitting in a classroom where a number of the participants suffered from a chronic illness or had relatives so afflicted. The general consensus seemed to be that they were tired of hearing people say, "Oh, I heard about a cure for your problem," or "You can cure that with diet." Just the trauma of living through the situation was enough; they did not need the meddling.

I thought for a long time about that conversation. There are several reasons, in my opinion, for this often-unsolicited advice:

1) People are very uncomfortable around those who are suffering from an illness, a disability, or a major life's trauma. If they can feel helpful by offering an idea that just might work, they do not feel so helpless. Like a barn-raising or quilting bee, people want to help their neighbors—and we are all neighbors.

2) If someone has some experience with a particular problem, he or she might want to offer to others any expertise that they may have gained. We all get advice from our friends such as how to get strawberry juice out of a white blouse, how often to change the oil in the car, and so on. This is part of the human experience, part of our culture.

3) People care. They want to help, and they want to give of themselves. They see this advice as part of that help. For centuries, we have helped where we could with our

neighbors. Help is how this country, indeed the socialized world, was created.

I can speak from the experience of being on the receiving end of some of this helpful advice, from acupuncture to bee stings. And, of course, there is my mother, who asks me every week if I have taken brewers yeast. I don't think we can afford to overlook anyone's well-intentioned ideas. Of course, we must avoid jumping at the latest "cure" announced these days on the Internet. We must use common sense, but we owe our friends and loved ones (even the meddling ones) a great debt of gratitude for caring.

I think that we need to understand the reasons that people offer advice and accept it graciously. I know it gets on your nerves, but it isn't really difficult just to say "thank you" to well-meaning friends and family members. Relationships are very important in our lives. We need them even more when we are challenged than other times because we have less security in our lives. You may not agree with me, as some of my classmates did not, but I think that the least we can do is to listen and accept help or advice in the spirit with which it is given. And we should be glad for friends and family who have that spirit.

CHAPTER 7

A POSITIVE MENTAL ATTITUDE WILL OVERCOME EVEN THE WORST HARDSHIP

Yes, it works! When I took the Dale Carnegie course, we used an exercise that had us chant "act enthusiastic, and you will be enthusiastic" over and over again. Haven't you ever noticed that when you "put on a happy face" you start to cheer yourself up? My objective in this book is to help you enjoy the only life you will get, so why not look at it with a positive attitude? Does complaining get you further? I doubt it. People react better to positive people and want to be around them. Any book on success will tell you to surround yourself with successful people, and most of these people got there with a positive attitude about their job, their accomplishments and their relationships.

While I was writing this book, my doctor, Gail Campofiore, asked me if I could include what gives some people the ability to withstand physical hardships, while others cannot. I did a little research for her, and discovered that there is such a thing as "hardiness." This is a syndrome marked by commitment, challenge and control that is purportedly associated with strong stress resistance. Hardy subjects tend to appraise potentially stressful events as less threatening than others do.[14] Research also suggests that optimists cope with stress in more adaptive ways than pessimists, and are likely to engage in more action-oriented, problem-focused copying. Some of the research my sister just finished at Pennsylvania State University dealt with the

---

[14] Brooks & Cole, **Psychology**.

fact that people are under more stress when they have less control over their environment. So, it stands to reason that taking control over your own adaptation to your situation, whether it be to change professions, go back to school, or go to counseling, gets you off on a path more likely to lead to success.

A positive mental attitude means not only that you see life in a positive manner, but that you set goals to help you get there. With a goal, you have to "see the winning." When I used to jog, I set a goal and could see that finish line. When I was going through graduate school, I could see that cap and gown. I heard a story some years ago about a Navy POW in Viet Nam who could see himself on the golf course every day for the seven years he spent in captivity. He practiced his swing in his mind so many times that, upon being released, he played his goal the first time he played golf!

You may have seen the movie "Born on the 4th of July," based on the life of Viet Nam veteran Ron Kovac. Ron had to work long and hard to meet his goals and make the difference he intended. He had a terrible disability to overcome. But many thousands of people are benefiting from his activism and his vision of what he wanted from his life.

Earlier I mentioned George and Tena Baehm, the "little people" who have given me so much inspiration. Their positive attitude toward life and toward other people creates a magnet that draws other people to them. They believe and practice that "life is what you make it." An aunt told George that he could be as successful as he wanted to be. Over the years he has proven her prediction by running his family business. You cannot go away from a conversation with Tena and George without feeling very lucky that you know these people!

A few pages back, I mentioned Greg Smith, the wheelchair bound talk show host in Phoenix, Arizona. Greg has his own little speech when his kids need something to pick them up: "So shall a man believe in himself; if you have a will and that will is strong, you can be strong. Think positively and never dwell on the negative." Having read many accounts of people like this in my research, I know that a common trait for people who have overcome difficult challenges is a positive mental attitude about themselves and their opportunities.

I know that I can change my mood by just putting on a Zig Ziglar tape, or Frank Sinatra music. You may be what you eat, but you are also what you think, and you are in total control of that.

My students hear from me every semester that employers are looking for "attitude and the ability to communicate" in their employees. This has not changed since I started teaching. Your attitude is important in getting a job, keeping a job, and most importantly in living your life.

As I write these words, Bill Clinton is President of the United States. His mother, the late Virginia Kelly, was a model of the value of a positive mental attitude. Virginia Kelly's life contained ample tragedy—"poverty, widow's veils, cancer, the arrest of her youngest son, Roger, on drug charges.... yet in the darkest moments she stubbornly refused to adopt a gloomy mind, insisting to all that the secret to life was to take whatever happened and just keep going."[15]   The press has always been quick to report on Virginia Kelly's spirit, and the fact that she would pump up everyone in campaign headquarters when things looked the darkest. "She was, perhaps, the world's greatest optimist", said Richard Mintz, a former campaign official.[16] Virginia Kelley had no special training, no college education to teach her how to battle cancer, how to get on with her life after the rough times struck. She used incredible talent to warm the hearts of those around her. She used a positive mental attitude to wring the most from her life and to give the most to those for whom she cared.

One of the most incredible examples of positive mental attitude comes from the wife of one of the Los Angeles MS Board Members, Melva Green. She was diagnosed in 1959 with Multiple Sclerosis, as a new bride. When I see Melva now, forty-two years later, I am always amazed and humbled that she keeps a smile on her face despite almost total immobility. In 1969, she wrote an article for the National Multiple Sclerosis Society, Southern California Chapter[17], in which she said the following: "I, like most MS patients, even those much worse than I, am very cheerful and optimistic and give thanks to God for the many blessings He has bestowed on me, the two most important being my eternal faith in Him, and my wonderful husband to share that faith with me. In another part of the article, Melva explores the disadvantage of not having a positive attitude: "would you harbor self pity and become impossible to live with, so that even the best husband would be forced to leave

---

[15] Lauter, D. "Virginia Kelley, Clinton's Mother, Dies at age 70." *The Los Angeles Times*, January 7, 1994.

[16] Ibid.

[17] Green, M. "MS and I." National Multiple Sclerosis Society, 1969.

you, and you therefore become miserable?" I know that many marriages could use her example, whether or not one partner suffers from a physical challenge.

Jimmie Heuga took third place in the slalom at the 1964 Winter Olympics. His reaction to his MS was to look at the problem as a challenge. He founded the Jimmie Heuga Center for the Reanimating of the Physically Challenged. In his words, "The key thing is motivation; it's impossible for us to care more about the participant's health than they do. Taking charge means working to do what I have always done: lead a very active life." Jimmie does not deny the reality but uses his knowledge to push himself and others toward better health.

Everyone wants to be successful, whether it is as a gardener, parent or corporation president. The elements are not difficult to understand. Disabilities and other challenges often give people the excuse to feel they do not need to succeed because of their problems. But you can see from the above list that everyone can be successful at something--and that something is their choice.

Valerie Slimp is certainly not using any excuses to keep herself from being an incredible role model. A quadruple amputee because of a rare infection possibly due to an insect bite, this woman, who has two children, is stopping at nothing to live a normal life. Her attitude is remarkable; yet she says, "I don't see myself as a blessing. A role model, maybe, because I DID survive this. Maybe now I can help others. I can be a sounding board." I was amazed to read her story, and I am sure you will agree that her positive mental attitude has helped her a great deal in her daily challenges.

Can you imagine selling orange juice for a living? At least you know that Ed Bahara, the Regional Sales Manager for Vita-Pakt Citrus Products in Los Angeles, rarely gets a cold! Ed shared his story with me and explained how much a positive mental attitude has had to do with his recovery. Ed spent nearly a year in a Long Beach hospital due to a fall that caused extensive brain damage. Although Ed stressed the need for patience and commitment to getting better, he also mentioned several times that "Every week gets better." I am convinced, as I am sure Norman Cousins would be, that Ed is getting better in part because of his attitude and commitment.

Do not be a victim. "Woe is me" is heard all too often when speaking to those afflicted with one problem or another. Everyone has problems, and there is always someone with greater problems than yours.

A victim is powerless, but none of us is really powerless. As I have said before and will say again, we all have choices about how we control our lives. If you use your personal strength to manage and create the things you can do, you will not feel like a victim and you will not act like one either. People who use their power are much more likely to engender support for their causes and their needs because they do not act like "victims". Every book I have ever read about people who overcame adversity includes references to the activist role they have taken, whether it is to start a self-help group or get funding to help themselves and others. Thousands of people die of AIDS every year, but those who are most involved with managing their illness have a better outcome.

I have a very close friend whose MS forced her to retire from teaching after eighteen years. Every once in a while, she talks about going back to teaching because she has much to offer in the classroom. But she insists, "I won't teach in a wheelchair." All of the examples I give her of people who do just that fail to change her mind. She prefers to let her disability keep her from making the kind of contribution she is so well qualified to make. I respect her choice but know that she has so much to offer in terms of her experience in the classroom.

The "victim" mentality says "The world owes me a living." Why not take advantage of disability payments if I can? Why work to better myself or get an education if the state will pay me to stay home? The welfare program in this country was designed to protect widows from the First World War, who had no other means of support because federal programs for military casualties had not been created yet. Yet, now it seems to protect many people who choose to be victims of their own behavior, such as alcoholism, or unwed parenthood. It costs one percent of our federal budget. One percent may not seem like much, until you figure that the Federal Budget is several trillion dollars! This is part of the reason that, when my doctor and my employer suggested that I apply for disability retirement, I refused. Why should I do that, I asked my doctor? "Your insurance company will pay for it," he said. No, it is that kind of victim mentality that decreases the total amount of productivity possible in the workforce. No one owes me a living. It is not the state's responsibility to pay for my lost wages. It is my responsibility to be flexible enough to retrain myself. When manufacturing companies move their facilities offshore to save money, there is often a major labor problem because the manufacturing employees do not have the skills to do anything else. If the Internet revolution has taught us anything, it is the necessity to upgrade our skills. Our only job security is the value of our skills, and that is no-one's responsibility but ours. One example is the decline in defense jobs in Southern California several years ago. Fifty thousand managers lost their jobs a month, and the real estate market tanked. What happened? Within three years, all those jobs had been recreated in the entertainment, software and healthcare industries. Those people who looked at their skills with the flexibility to survive this kind of industrial revolution are alive and thriving today.

Earlier I mentioned Norman Cousins' book **Head First**. In it he mentions several examples of people who seemed to have recovered remarkably because they chose to fight and not give in to a diagnosis. They chose to pursue their options and, when needed, became flexible.

Doctors are continuing to find some correlation between adaptive emotional attitudes and a better immune system. So much for letting oatmeal take the credit! In addition to Dr. Bernie Siegal and Norman Cousins, there has been and continues to be, much research into the mind-body connection between disease, the immune system, and the mind. "Scientists have shown that mental states such as stress and depression have a clear influence on the immune system….hinting that psychological and social approaches may have an important role to play in preventing disease or shortening its course. Indeed, recent studies of people with a range of illnesses from the common cold to AIDS strongly suggest that a greater emphasis on emotion and attitudes could serve the public health and save the nation money….these and similar research projects herald an important new era, in which the mind will be recognized as being equally important as the body in the practice of medicine," said Susan Blumenthal, chief of preventive and behavioral medicine at the National Institute of Mental Health."[18] This information supports my lifelong theory: If you "act enthusiastic," you can "be enthusiastic." There is more evidence than can possibly be included here, but the scientific experiments surrounding everything from using pets in eldercare to using clowns in hospitals point to the priceless benefits of a positive mental attitude.

I have a number of posters in my office with motivational sayings and letters on them. One of them is of a bicyclist riding on a country road, head down. "You must believe to achieve," it says. It reminds me of a quote from **Think and Grow Rich**, by Napolean Hill: "Anything you can believe, you can achieve." But you have to believe it first!

The first time my husband and I attempted to ride in a bike tour to benefit the Multiple Sclerosis Society, nine years ago, I had to believe I could do it, or I would have given up! Scared? You bet! But I could see the winning, see the finish line. When everyone else told me not to try to ride the bike because I might fall off, I told them I would risk the bruises and went on to complete the tour. Not without a few bruises, but I did finish! We trained every weekend on a tandem bike, and I gradually increased my strength. What was the worst that could happen? You truly must believe that you can do it to achieve it.

Jerry Deets is a Santa Cruz wheelchair road racer who definitely feels that he has much to offer and a much to teach. "I can do anything anybody else can do. I might be a little

[18] Weiss, R. "Linking physical and emotional health." *The Washington Post,* January 11, 1994.

slower, but there's nothing I can't do. That's why it's important for me to be looked at as an athlete." When it comes to hills, Jerry just keeps pushing!

Achievement is Disney's middle name! Who among us has not delighted at the philosophy on which Walt Disney built his business? Pat Williams, the Orlando Magic basketball-team manager, quotes the secrets of Disney and how they cut across everything we do:

> *Make tomorrow pay off today*
> *Free the imagination*
> *Build with lasting quality in mind*
> *Fortitude and perseverance*
> *HAVE FUN!*[19]

Any Disney employee is trained to use a positive attitude to make sure all visitors have a good time. Why not use that philosophy in living our lives as well! I know that I learned the importance of a positive attitude while I was participating in one of the research projects at UCLA, where I went once a week for an injection of an experimental drug. One of the nurses wore a button that read: "Enjoy life. This is not a dress rehearsal." I commented on it and she gave me one, which I am proud to wear whenever possible. As I have been saying, and will continue to say, we have only one chance at this marvelous experience called life, and it's up to us to make the best use of it.

---

[19] Pat Williams, Orlando Magic basketball team manager.

Through my association with the Multiple Sclerosis Society, I have become acquainted with Dr. Wallace Tourtellotte, chief of neurological services at the VA Medical Center in West Los Angeles. Dr. Tourtellotte carries around all sorts of sayings meant to put a smile on your face. I would like to share one of his aphorisms with you now:

Happiness is an attitude
Happiness is found along the way, not at the journey's end.
Get past mad fast!
Positive attitude changes everything!
The heart that gives...gathers

Dr. Tourtellote is a true scientist who gives of himself so that the lives of his patients may be better. My life is always better when I am in his presence.

During the six years that I was studying for my Ph.D., I was putting together ideas for my dissertation. An original plan for my hypothesis was that there is a relationship between attitude and customer satisfaction; in other words, the better the attitude of the waitress, car attendant or telephone operator, the better the experience for the customer and the more likely he or she will come back. I know this seems elementary to you, but it is amazing how many services fail to invest time into training their people to display the proper attitude. A positive mental attitude can help anyone do a better job! It can most certainly help you to have a better life!

As I said in the last chapter, you can do anything you want if you take it "one step at a time." I am POSITIVE that I will continue to live my life to the fullest? Why not? It sure beats the alternative.

CHAPTER 8

WHAT DO YOU HAVE TO LOSE?

Twenty years ago, I was a sales trainer for a bank. I trained customer service representatives to "sell" bank services such as checking accounts, lines of credit, etc. Prior to that time, banks had not done much sales training and the customer service representatives found the prospect of setting *GOALS* to cross-sell various services frightening. What if they didn't reach the goal? What if they only sold 15% instead of 25% and reached only 40% of their goal? I asked them, "Didn't you accomplish more by setting the goal than you would have without it?" In other words, if they had not set the goal or embarked on this program, they might not have sold any checking accounts! I asked them what they had to lose by setting the goal. They would most certainly sell something and be able to improve their results with each month. And they most certainly did-by over 100%!

The first time I ran a 10K race, I knew I would not win it, but what did I have to lose by entering? I had only to gain in experience, good health and motivation to run another one. And, of course, I gained the t-shirt from the event!

What do you have to lose by setting a goal to take a course, to get involved in a support group, to add a skill that prepares you for a different career? The worst that can happen is that you will not complete the goal that particular time, but you just set another goal and try again. Most people make decisions based on the chance of the outcome being better than if they did not attempt the task. When I bought that exercise video, I knew that the risk was small-the risk of wasting the $20 that the video cost. Sure, I might fall as well, but that's old news around our house! The risk was worth it.

It works that way in the stock market. You invest in stocks because the chances are better that you will make money by investing than by the alternative of not investing or by investing in something else. You take a job because the chances are better that you will be happier with the job than if you stayed where you were.

I recently had a friend ask me if she should consider learning to sky dive. I asked her what was the worst that could happen? She could die. Was she willing to take the chance? If so, she should learn to sky dive. She told me that no one had put it in those terms before, but it put the responsibility in her hands, and she felt good about that.

So what do you have to lose if you are confined to a Wheelchair, and you decide to enter a marathon? The worst that can happen is that you will tip over or not get very far. So what? A few scratches, a bruised ego, but you can always try again.

When I teach personal selling or produce corporate sales seminars, I love to talk about the worst that can happen if you ask for the order. The person to whom you are trying to sell will say no. Or he/she might kick you out of the office. Here I speak from experience! But the prospect will not take out a gun and shoot the salesman. I will admit that it is easy for me to write about this because I have had twenty-five years of facing rejection in the field of selling. I have had to learn not to take it personally, but to get up and go back in the ring. What was most critical for me was to learn not to take rejection personally, and to try again.

As I am now responsible for the undergraduate marketing program at The University of La Verne, I find myself taking all kinds of risks to bring new courses to the program when I am not sure we will get the number of students required to offer the courses. What is the worst that can happen? I will get fired? Well, I have been fired before; and, besides, I was looking for a job when I found this one! Seriously, I find that calculated risks, with as much information as possible before decisions are made, are the most likely to move us ahead in the long run.

So what do you have to lose? A little time, maybe, a little pride, maybe? Whatever happens, you will have learned something. But most of us have the time to start over and can muster the energy to reset the goal. Life is like a tree that grows branches in a variety of ways--you just have to be able to switch the branches as your needs and desired goals require.

So, what do you have to lose? And don't you have more to gain?

CHAPTER 9

IMPROVE ON THE WORST THAT CAN HAPPEN

For many of you, a disability is the worst that can happen. But preparing for your future is productive and puts you in a position to control your life.

Suppose that losing your job is the worst that can happen now. What will you do then? Find another, change careers, sell your home, sell some investments? When we bought our present home, I was afraid to make such a large investment because of the high mortgage. My father gave me some of the best advice I have ever been given: "What is the worst that can happen, and what will you do if it does?" It was a good question. We thought that losing our jobs was the worst that could happen (the innocence of youth and good health). So we decided that we would have to sell some stock that my father had given me when he retired from Westinghouse. Well we both lost our jobs within the first three years of owning the house. But we made it through and did not have to sell the stock. As you probably know, 99% of the things you worry about will never happen. But at least we were prepared. I honestly think that preparing for the worst that can happen gives you a great deal of peace of mind.

Because I suffer from a progressive illness, I am preparing for the worst that can happen to me. This gives me control, gives me more options and allows me to accept situations that may arise. I encourage everyone to prepare and improve on the worst that can happen. An education can give you choices and open doors, no matter what the disability! As a matter of fact, an education gives you choices all by itself, even if you never face the kind of challenges I am discussing here. I have a cube of writing paper in my office that is inscribed, "Think education is expensive? Try ignorance." Investing in those choices will be the best investment you ever made.

The next step to accepting the worst that can happen is to improve upon it. Some examples:

*The worst that can happen is you lose your job due to your disability. How do you turn this lemon into lemonade? You can look at alternatives that do not require the skill you no longer have. In my case, teaching does not require that I be able to walk. Telephone-heavy professions are a possibility. So are jobs that require driving but can adapt to wheelchair accessible vans. There are jobs for everyone who really wants one, believe me.

*The worst that can happen is you go blind. Although accepting that is probably the hardest thing you have ever done, how can you improve upon it? I once saw a movie about a library employee who was blind--but the library patrons did not know it. This employee gave information and directions completely, to the satisfaction of her employer and to her own fulfillment. She may have been doing something different than she would otherwise have chosen, but she had improved on the "worst that can happen."

*The worst that can happen to you is you lose the use of your arms. I not only have read books written about or by people in this situation, but I also have a friend who typed with her chin in a Morse-code type of function. Let me tell you a little more about Geri Esten. Geri, who passed away in 1996 at the age of 49, had not had the use of her arms and legs for over fifteen years; yet she insisted on living independently. By independently, I mean that she had a caregiver, but she was not in a nursing home or other care facility. Geri "figured out" that she did not want that type of lifestyle. Her doctor recommended that she go into a nursing home, but Geri persisted in her desire to continue to live in Venice, California. Can you imagine becoming a licensed Marriage and Family Counselor with that many strikes against you? Geri continued to educate herself and, at one point, could not take a course in linguistics in which she was interested only because the class was full! When I last visited Geri, she showed me some of the things that she could do with her computer. I wish you could have seen her face light up when she talked about how "neat" it was! The computer opened up all sorts of opportunities for her. She improved on the "worst" with the use of a computer, and she has written me letter-perfect correspondence with it!

Actually, folks, the worst that can happen is that you lose your life. And it won't make any difference whether you accept that or not. Anything else can be improved upon with a little ingenuity, support and belief in possibilities.

CHAPTER 10

RELAX

I wish I had a nickel for all the times someone has told me to relax in my life. I happen to be a Type A personality, always moving and never able to sit still. Patience is also not one of my virtues. I cannot even watch much television because I keep wondering what else I could be doing that would be more productive. But I am trying to change that. Maybe it is reaching my forties or maybe it is paying attention to my own "smell the roses" plaque in the living room.

Life is terrific, as far as I am concerned. I am taking more time to smell those roses, to appreciate "people watching" and to be more patient with the crowded world in which we live. When I was traveling a great deal, my job frequently put me in situations where unavoidable delays produced raw nerves among travelers. I have learned that, unless I have the responsibility for flying the plane, I will not worry about it and just RELAX. Of course, I did prepare for "the worst that can happen" if I missed that meeting; but, once I had done all I could to control the situation, I am happy to say that I relaxed. What a wonderful past time to discover! I got such joy from watching small children discover the wonders of flying rather than worrying about my next appointment. This attitude really helped during one of the semesters when I was teaching sales management at California Polytechnic University in Pomona, California. I was in San Antonio, Texas after calling on our largest customer. The plane from San Antonio to Dallas was delayed, which meant that I would miss the connection to

Ontario, and thus the class I was supposed to teach at 6:30. I called the school, asked them to put a note on the door, and went back to whatever I was doing. The outcome of missing the class would have been the same whether I wasted time fretting over it or not. Because I did not, I made good use of the waiting time rather than wasting an opportunity to get more reading done. And I probably do not need to tell you that students are not exactly heartbroken when class is canceled!

Life is much easier for you "Type B" people! Being able to take life as it comes instead of trying to force it makes the roses smell even sweeter!

When I teach sales management, I use Dale Carnegie's book, **How to Stop Worrying and Start Living.** Although he writes much about "the worst that can happen," Carnegie quotes many people who wrapped themselves up in their worry to the point that they thought they were going to die. Only then did they relax and accept their fate. Guess what happened? They got better! Fully one-third of corporate executives come down with diseases like ulcers, heart trouble and high blood pressure because they let the stress of their job affect their physical being! I have Dale Carnegie to thank for changing my view of my life, and I will be forever grateful for what he has given me. Of course, relaxing is even more difficult in our world of "instant communication," via cell phones, beepers, and email. But you have the power to use these conveniences and not to let them use you.

Relaxing also helps you concentrate. I use an exercise in my class where the students sit quietly and count to ten over and over again. They try not to let their minds wander-- if they do, they bring them back again to one ...two....three....

Doing this exercise for 20 minutes each morning has helped me concentrate and relax before important public speaking engagements.

Meditation is a thousands-of-years-old technique for concentration and communication. Books and classes about meditation never seem to go out of favor. Maybe in this world where people have less and less free time every year, meditation can help them relax. No matter what method works for you, there are many from which to choose.

Very often, when I am overwhelmed with responsibilities that have to be done 'today', I take a deep breath and use my time management techniques to pick out the most important one that has to be done 'right now'. That deep breath is a way of relaxing and putting things into perspective. If you have two or three important things to do, such as the laundry, write a letter, or pay the bills, you can prioritize which one has to be accomplished right now and move one from there. Making those kinds of choices gives you control and helps you accomplish more.

Remember, we all have a very short time on this grand earth. We can get the most out of it if we relax and enjoy it!

Relax and "hang in there." You have everything to gain!

CHAPTER 11

KEEP YOUR SENSE OF HUMOR

Very important!

There is nothing funny about a disability or a major challenge, but dealing with it by using a sense of humor can make life easier for you and for those with whom you live or work. It can remove some of the difficulty from a tense situation. Remember the cartoonist, John Callahan, in Oregon? That is part of what he does to help his readers find humor wherever they can. And my "little people" friends George and Tena Baehm use their sense of humor to delight their friends and others they meet. When George asks help in his business, and someone tells him that they are "short-handed today," he reminds them that he is always short-handed!

In my family, we find that kidding about some of the things that happen to me helps us to get through them. M y husband likes to prod me about a block from home with the comment, "you might as well start getting out of the car now; it takes you so long!" Although I know he would coddle me if I wanted him to, making jokes about the "jobs" I can no longer do (believe me, I don't miss taking out the trash!) keeps things light. At the trade shows I used to work, my colleagues loved to ride the Amigo I used. It is much easier to make jokes about it than to cry about it! As a matter of fact, I credit humor as a major part of the enjoyment John and I receive from our marriage.

And so it goes. You may be saying "This is ridiculous; why would you laugh about a thing like that?" Why not? Does it do you any good to curse the fates every time you fall or can't do something you want? Sawing sawdust does not correct the wrong.

Norman Cousins spent much of his life researching the effect of humor on seriously ill patients. He found that remarkable results were accomplished when funny movies were shown--remarkable physical effects!

If you will look through history or happen to follow politics, you will find that humor is used to break the ice in many tense situations. It is also one of the most important techniques used by public speakers. I am also positive that you have noticed the tendency to use humor by disabled people who have made an effort to live their lives to the fullest.

Last year, several well-meaning friends gave me a calendar "For Women Who Do Too Much." Each day has a special quote designed to make the owner of the calendar feel like everything is not falling apart! On March 26th,1993, the following entry caught my eye: *"Good humor is very inexpensive. It is one of the pleasures in life that is relatively free. I'm sure if we try hard enough, we can remember a part of us that used to laugh and be playful. I'm sure it's still there somewhere."*

By the way, did you know that you create fewer lines in your face from laughing than from frowning? Many fewer lines!

So, now you know that "the best things in life" really are free! I like to concentrate on productive ways to live my life, and I find that laughing makes my life more productive than crying. Try it.

CHAPTER 12

CONCENTRATE ON RELATIONSHIPS

Although I've spent a lot of my business career striving to reach my business goals, I am lucky to have developed some wonderful friendships along the way and to have kept in touch with my family. If someone were to ask me what I consider successful about my career, I would have to answer the long-term friendships I have developed because they are worth more than any short-term order for product. I am fortunate to be able to spend much of the Christmas holidays calling some of the people I used to work with all over the country, and to relive those wonderful relationships.

In 1992, Barbara Bush spoke to the graduates of Wellesley College. Although her appearance was protested by some as inappropriate because, in their opinion, she had not accomplished anything of note on her own, I think she made an important point. She said that the relationships you have would be what are important to you in years to come, not your grades today. When my students become overly concerned about their grades or "what is on the exam," I put forth this comment as one of the most important I have heard in my life. If you really think about the importance of the relationships you have developed during your life, both with family and friends, I think you'll agree with me.

Remember the theme of this book--to live your life fully, whatever your hardships. Wheelchairs do not restrict friendships and families are incredibly supportive when given the chance. I am so fortunate to have a wonderful family because they give me the strength to overlook my condition and concentrate on what is good about my life--believe me, my family and my husband top that list.

In Los Angeles, as I imagine in other cities, we have psychologists on the radio in the afternoon. On holidays, when I have been in the kitchen preparing the Thanksgiving or Christmas meal, I have listened to these shows and been amazed at the petty situations and confrontations that have caused years of estrangement between family members. People harbor grudges for years and miss out on relationships that will enrich their lives. You can never get the time back that you lost by not speaking to that brother-in-law or other family member. The last thing you want is to feel guilty at a funeral for refusing to mend those fragile fences. I can attest to this mistake personally, because I said something to my mother-in-law many years ago that so distressed her that she did not speak to me for two years. The point was not whether I was right or not (I just wanted to be around more positive people at that time in my life and was tired of her complaining); the point was that the remark caused pain to my husband and his mother for a long time. It was definitely not worth being right. That was one of those instances where you can win the battle and lose the war. I hope I learned that lesson well.

I recently heard a radio psychologist begin his daily program on KABC radio with the following appropriate comment: "Make the important things in life take the time they deserve." Because life is so hectic these days and people move so frequently, relationships take work to keep. But, they are worth it. Sometimes you have to put into perspective how you are spending your time. A simple phone call can bring all sorts of new opportunities. I have a good friend who is the president of a large corporate division in my former business. He takes time every Christmas to call his best customers just to wish them a happy holiday. Nothing more. That is relationship building!

Cherish your relationships. They are gold and are the very fiber of life.

CHAPTER 13

WHAT IS YOUR CHOSEN METHOD FOR CONTRIBUTING TO LIFE?

We are sometimes caught up in attributing our "being" to what we do for a living. I recently heard a friend in a counseling session refer to himself as "an old man and a cripple." That is certainly not the way I see him! Just because he does not work does not mean that he is not contributing to society, whether it is as a husband, father, grandfather or volunteer counselor.

When I lost my job several years ago, I made the mistake of thinking my contribution to society was tied up in my profession. But I learned quickly that I was valued for what I had done in my life, not just for that job. I cherish the letter from a student who told me how much impact I had on her life. I will certainly cherish that letter more than the last one million dollar order I wrote! That letter was also the most important contributor to my decision to pursue the field of education as my second career.

Dr. Joyce Brothers says that the way we dress, the occupation we choose, the mate we select, our moral conduct--all these things--are tied to the picture we have of ourselves. We are all unique and different. We all have abilities and talents. When one ability is taken away, we, and only we, have the chance to substitute another one.

What do you do?

Who are you?

Most of us answer these questions with what other people think we are or pay us to be. But is your answer what is most important to you? Perhaps now is the time to take a look at what you want that answer to be.

One of the books I use in the Sales Management course I teach is called **How to Get Control of Your Time and Your Life**, by Alan Lakein. One of the most important chapters (at least to most of my students) deals with goals-- what do you want to accomplish in the next year, in three years and in five years? Along with this exercise, the students must answer what they would be doing if they only had six months to live. Moral? If you are not working on long-term goals now, take another look at your goals.

So you have a disability that prevents you from building houses or running marathons or typing manuscripts--well, that is not all you were or are. Or you are grieving the loss of a mate of many years. Your function as a wife, mother, husband, and so on has only been part of your life. You are now charged with the task of using your remaining abilities and relationships to get the most from your life. Sawing sawdust ("I used have so much fun when Joe was alive") is useless. We all have a marvelous capacity to enjoy a variety of experiences in our lives. Just because one of those experiences no longer fits into your bag does not mean you reduce what you do or who you are--you just re-arrange it a bit! I used to do much sewing and cooking, primarily because I was married to a musician who worked every weekend and left me with time to pursue these activities. My life is different today, with different priorities. Frankly, the lack of strength in my right hand would not allow me to do much sewing, and moving around the kitchen is too difficult to pursue those cookie marathons any more. Do I feel a little guilty for not producing hundreds of Christmas cookies? Sure, maybe out of some nostalgia, but I am no less of a valuable person because I do not produce a freezer full of goodies. My life is different, but no less fulfilling. When people ask me if I made the cookies I am serving now, I laugh and say "Yes, I made the money that bought them." Thankfully, our lives today do not require many of the domestic chores some of our mothers had to contend with. I can go down to the local market and pick up a fully cooked turkey dinner. My friends will appreciate it because, after all, we get together for the company and not the food, and I will have a better time. Not a high price to pay for gravy that is not lumpy!

What is the only thing that gives you absolutely unconditional love? That does not turn its back on you when you fall down or get fired or make a mistake? Your dog, of course. Your dog makes his contribution to you by being there, by loving you. That is what dogs do, that is their contribution to life, security considerations notwithstanding. I do not ask of my husband that he buy me gifts in order to be loved and I do not call my mother on Sunday because I have to. These people are valuable to me for who and what they are. Life can be so simple if we look at how we want to contribute, what resources we want to use, and concentrate on what we do well and want to do.

I am familiar with a widow who asked the question "What is the meaning of life?" after her husband passed away. Why are we on this earth? To live! The meaning of life lies within us all, not within anyone or anything else. Although you have the responsibility to choose the way you live your life, you also have the freedom.

I am also familiar with the vice president of marketing for a large company in the home center industry who recently underwent surgery for brain cancer. We talked about his current responsibilities and the choices he is making. He said, " My philosophy is either you can sit on your ass and feel sorry for yourself or you can do all that you can to make the people around you feel comfortable, and that things are business as usual. I chose the option that works for me." His colleagues do not only admire Bob, but he has all the support he needs from his family and friends. That is the way he has chosen to live his life.

Just because you have a disability does not mean that you cannot reach your goals, whatever they may be. It may be tougher, but it can still be done. One of the members of my Toastmasters group recently gave a speech about a World War II pilot with no legs! After he lost his legs in an accident, the Air Force discharged him. But the war opened up an opportunity for him to fulfill his goals—to fly bombers. When he was captured by the Germans, he found out that he was famous!

Peter Dawson is an excellent example of what can be done. He is a blind attorney in Seattle, Washington. Comments made about him include the following: "He will pursue something until there is nothing left to pursue". He has found answers that have changed laws for the betterment of people. During his legal training, Peter learned to rely on his intelligence, where formerly he relied on athletic prowess. He even skis, with one of his five brothers coaching him through a headset.

Dr. Phil McDonough has chosen to use his talents to further the causes of disabled people everywhere. His passion once was restoring Ford Mustangs. When he could not do that anymore, he said, "okay, don't sit around!" He channels his energies into teaching and consulting.

I am spending more time in volunteer activities for the Multiple Sclerosis Society and other motivational activities because that is the way I have chosen to contribute to life. Sure, I value my job and intend to continue, but my value as a person is not tied up in my job alone. Nor is it tied up in Christmas cookies! I realize that we have too short a time on earth to waste it in activities that do not benefit ourselves and other people. I think my generation, the seventy-eight million baby boomers born between 1946 and 1964, has through the years thought we were what was written on our business cards. Many of us have learned the hard way to appreciate relationships and to realize that what we are may have very little to do with what is on our business cards.

A disability or an emotional challenge is enough of a crutch. I have little patience for people who use it to avoid their responsibility to live their life to the fullest. As I have been reminding you throughout this "journey," how you live your life is your choice, and the outcome either hurts or harms you.

Reach into your bag of "who I am"--you will find many tantalizing and exciting titles: parent, spouse, teacher, friend, committee member, church member, dishwasher, letter writer, companion, best friend, and on and on and on. The different road your life took has just as many branches and just as many possibilities--only different ones. Some doors have closed and others have opened.

A disability requires an adjustment in life, but it does nothing to one's value. What do you want to do with your life? Remember my earlier quote from Geri Esten: "Figure out what you want to do and do it."

I am reminded of the story of Rebecca Lukens. The wife of a steel mill owner in rural Pennsylvania during the 19th Century, Rebecca had four children and a big decision to make when her husband suddenly died. Rebecca decided, as I hope you will, that **IF IT IS TO BE, IT IS UP TO ME.** She knew that the responsibility for her happiness and her family's welfare lay in her hands, no one else's. Rebecca managed Luken's Steel as she and her husband had dreamed and intended to nurture it. Today Luken's Steel is a Fortune 500 company because Rebecca Lukens knew that **IF IT IS TO BE, IT IS UP TO ME.**

If you want excitement in your life, you have to create it because only you know what kind of excitement you want. In this country, we have some 250 million different people who want different things from their lives. Do not wait for someone else to create excitement for you because no one can do it as well as you can.

There may be nothing you can do about your disability or the incident that created the tough challenge you are now facing, but there is plenty you can do to reach your goals and support your desire to live your life to the fullest.

One of the seminars I do in our sales training company, Capital Associates, centers on what makes people successful. I would like to share it with you because I think you can relate this acronym to your own desire to be successful, with whatever limitations you have; also to your own definition of what success means in your life:

Strive to be Better

Understanding

Commitment to Excellence

Control

Enthusiasm

Sense of Purpose

Set Goals

Is there any one of these that does not apply to our challenge? If you work with this acronym for success, you will realize that success does require that you embrace excellence, that you understand others, that you control impulses to sway from your goals, that you adhere closely to your purpose and to your goals. No one is perfect not even the able-bodied. We all need to strive to be better at everything we do. Leila Josefewitz, a young violinist, practices many hours a day, even though she is already extremely accomplished. I used to strive to walk around the block every day. Most of the time, it was not very successful, but I always tried to improve on yesterday. Now that I am restricted to an exercise bike, I advance my time just a little every week.

I think we need to strive to improve our attitude every day, especially with a physical challenge. "Be the best that you can be" is used in advertisements for L'Oreal hair care products. Everyone can work on being the best and doing their best.

Understanding other people is part of getting through life successfully. Understand that

*People want to help.

*Everyone gets scared sometimes.

"Good enough is not enough" is one of the statements used in my seminars because mediocrity has overtaken much of America's attitudes. A commitment to excellence is the subject of many memos and articles about the manufacturing and service industries. We are in global competition every day of the week for business. When you say "Staying in bed today" is good enough for you, you are denying yourself the pleasure of getting (or being helped) out of bed.

Always strive for excellence in your life. Would putting a flower on your dinner tray turn it from a meal into a treat? Then do it! Always look for ways to delight yourself so that you can say, "I made an excellent day for myself!"

But sometimes things worth doing are worth doing badly. Does that make sense? Let me explain. Although I may say in my seminars "good enough is not enough," I am realistic to know that some things are better done less than perfectly than not done at all. An example might be the local bake sale. You cannot bake, but you can buy a contribution. Suppose you need to visit a relative in a nursing home, but have no money to bring a gift. I suspect that the visit alone will be a marvelous gift. A phone call can add much to a relationship, even when you would prefer to write a card. The important thing is to expand the options for achieving what you want, not to settle for second best.

Control and discipline are important contributors to meeting your challenges. If you discipline yourself to exercise every day or to read a chapter a day, you can have control over your life. Before her death, Geri Esten was in the process of writing a book about hiring and keeping caregivers. In this way, Geri was exercising control over her life.

I like to tell my classes that "Fifty percent of the sale is enthusiasm," and I firmly believe that. I have written earlier about enthusiasm and a positive mental attitude; so you should not be surprised to see it mentioned again. Zig Ziglar and Dale Carnegie consider enthusiasm a critical element for living life. To squeeze that last drop of pleasure out of today, try adding a spoonful of enthusiasm!

I have also spoken earlier about setting goals. In his book, **Over the Top**, Zig Ziglar mentions that academic literature confirms the fact that those who set goals perform better in a variety of tasks. On page 211, he mentions David Jensen, Chief Administrative Officer, Crump Institute of Biological Imaging for the UCLA School of Medicine. Mr. Jensen surveyed those who attend public seminars that Zig conducts around the country: He found that the goal setters earned more than twice what was earned by those who took no specific action to set their goals.

Are you are scratching your head and saying "What is she talking about? Goals! I have a hard enough time getting through the day!" So set a goal to "get through the day" with a smile on your face. Anybody can do that or set a goal to do the following

:

√ Save $2 a week   √ Read a book a month
√ Call a friend every day   √ Try a new exercise

It gives you control and the accomplishment is something to anticipate!

CHAPTER 14

TAKE CARE OF YOURSELF

No, this is not a lecture on the evils of cholesterol or coffee. It is just a comment that, regardless of the physical barriers to total functioning; taking care of yourself is always important. And, of course, that is your responsibility.

Zig Ziglar relates the story of the woman who lost her eyesight through a mistaken prescription and was awarded $1,000,000 by the insurance company, and of the man who lost the ability to walk after a plane crash and was also awarded $1,000,000. Would you give your eyesight for $1,000,000? Then it is best to appreciate what you do have. A disability does not mean that you are immune to other health problems. I wish it worked that way.

The modern world is rife with poisons and threats to our health. Yes, you do need to pay attention to good nutrition and exercise. What, you say? Don't I have enough problems being disabled? Is not this challenge of a divorce or the death of a loved one enough to bear? Well, because of your challenge, it is even more important to maximize your health so that you can deal in a more effective way with future challenges. I lost a very good friend several years ago, who was one of the most motivational people I have ever met. He handled his advancing multiple sclerosis with humor and courage. Unfortunately, when he died in an accident, they found advanced prostate cancer. No, we are not protected from any other challenges just because we already have plenty. Think of the biblical character Jobe, who was tested by losing much of what he cherished time and time again.

I know that I appreciate every day that I can navigate around my house or the grocery store because I do not know how long that will last. We all take for granted the ability to see, hear, talk, or whatever. Although I would not wish a disability on anyone, it does teach you to appreciate what you have left in a way that no one else can imagine.

I am not sure that George Burns was a model of physical fitness, but I know that he lived longer than most of us will; so he must have done something right! In his book **All My Best Friends** (Putnam, 1989), George alluded to getting older: "Some people get old better than others.....Look, it takes a lot of experience to grow old. I don't care how smart some of these younger kids are, it's going to take them a long time to learn how to do it. Because it takes a long time to get old. And you have to be very lucky. Look, I'll be very honest, being old is not the best thing that ever happened to me. But it's a great alternative." That is the trick! Recognize that being less than able-bodied is a great alternative to not being here at all! So when I say take care of yourself, I really mean take care of your mind, too. It can overcome and make less important many problems! Feeding your mind is just as important as feeding your body! Zig Ziglar admits that motivation, the kind you get from speakers and books, isn't permanent. But he also reminds us that bathing is not permanent either! We need to renew and refresh every day! Have you ever heard the saying, "today is the first day of the rest of your life?" That is even more reason to take care of whatever can help you start that road to the rest of your life in good condition. Zig is famous for reminding us to feed our minds as we feed our bodies.

I find that eating right and getting enough exercise are important parts of my overall health and add to my mental well-being. Want to know my secret? Grape Nuts® and oatmeal for breakfast! Here is the recipe: _ cup of each cereal, _ cup of skim milk, one minute and fifty seconds in the microwave. On TV, they advertise Grape Nuts with the invitation to "Try it for a week"; trust them, they are right! (No, I do not own stock in the corporate parent of Post Cereals!)

So take care of your million-dollar body and treat it like the temple that it is. It was given to you free, and all you have to do is maintain it, at very little cost considering its priceless worth. Good health will make it easier to face any challenge, any time.

CHAPTER 15

REMEMBER, YOU ALWAYS HAVE A CHOICE

The forefathers of this Country sometimes chose death over the deprivation of their liberty. It may not appear that you always have a choice, but you do.

You can accept your disability and try to improve upon it or you can express your anger to everyone who passes by. You can accept what created the challenge you are facing now (divorce, death, being fired from a job) and try to improve on it, or you can wallow in self-pity. The choice is entirely yours.

You can appreciate your relationships or decide that others must take care of you because they "owe you." You can find a career or avocation that pleases you, or you can decide that the world owes you a living. You do not have to dig too deeply into the history of the United States to know that the choices the revolutionary planners made were those that provided prosperity only if they created it themselves. Actually, George Washington probably made it a tougher choice when he told his soldiers that, if they won, he could not pay them, and they might starve; if they lost, they would be hung as traitors. My choices seem much easier when put in that context.

You can live the remainder of your life in darkness, brooding over your lot, or you can make the best of what you have and what you CAN do.

Franklin Roosevelt, who spent most of his life in a wheelchair, made that important choice--and aren't we glad he did!

Helen Keller made a remarkable choice to overcome the worst of disabilities and contributed remarkably to the world around her.

Abraham Lincoln said "People are about as happy as they make up their minds to be." It is true. You have the choice, perhaps not of your physical circumstances, but most certainly of how you react to them.

The choices you make today will affect the rest of your life; so make them carefully. The responsibility is yours, and the choice is yours.

John Stefancik and Craig Penniman had a choice. They could let their muscular dystrophy create barriers for them, or they could explore the Grand Teton National Park. Their choice certainly presented its challenges, for traveling facilities for the disabled traveler still present a number of problems. But Mr. Penniman knew that he would "only be able to travel for two or three more years because of his deteriorating condition...each day tests the group's stamina, but it is those moments-the flight of an osprey, a patch of wildflowers, a lone moose drinking from a mountain stream—that make the effort worthwhile."[20] Do you think they are glad they made that choice?

---

[20] Hirsch, J. "For disabled tourists, travel remains fraught with barriers, extra burdens." *The Wall Street Journal*, July 1, 1994.

CHAPTER 16

NEVER GIVE UP!

Forgive me as I put on my sales training hat--what are the five most important words leading to success at anything? In the words of Winston Churchill,

NEVER, NEVER, NEVER ....GIVE UP!

(I know, you peeked at the title of this chapter, but I wanted you to get the message fast!).

Wilma Rudolph did not give up. Stricken with polio at the age of four, the little girl from a large family in Tennessee faced life without the use of her crippled leg. But her mother did not give up. She massaged Wilma's leg, enlisting the help of the other children, for over two years. Wilma then used a brace for a time and finally discarded it. The sport Wilma chose was running! Although she displayed an unusual gait, her coach saw something special. In the 1956 Olympics, Wilma won a bronze medal in the 100 meter relay. Great, you say, for a young woman who was told she might never walk. Well, tuck this into your list of examples--in the 1960 Olympics, Wilma Rudolph won three gold medals. THREE GOLD MEDALS!! Why? Because Wilma's mother never gave up, Wilma never gave up and her coach gave support to her special spirit. Every time she failed, she came back again. I have no doubt that this is the secret of rehabilitation for more successful people than I could ever name here.

Michael Rilenge did not give up. He tried twice, and failed twice, to climb Mount McKinley. "So he did the next best thing. He climbed a mountain that's even taller..."On Saturday, February 25, 1995, Rilenge returned from a trip to the top of Aconcagua in Argentina, the highest peak in the Western Hemisphere. "It's just a dream," Rilenge said of his mountain climbing. "I'm just a normal guy with a dream. And muscular distrophy.... Rilenge said he climbs pretty much like anybody else, except he moves a little slower and the other members of his team are roped much closer to him than on a conventional climb.[21]" Although Rilenge credits his team with much of his success, the fact is that Michael Rilenge did not give up. In the face of a disability with which most people would not consider a sport such as mountain climbing, Micheal Rilenge did not give up. He knew that eventually he would make it. See the winning. He did that, I am sure, many times. And he made it.

Marilyn Bartlett has struggled for years to become a lawyer. She has failed the bar exam five times[22]. Looking back on my own struggle to earn my Ph.D., I know that most of us would have given up after that much disappointment. But this 49-year-old college professor, who suffers from dyslexia, recently won an important legal victory for people with learning disabilities. A federal judge in New York ordered the New York State Board of Law Examiners to give her twice the normal amount of time to take the test and other special accommodations that she requested under the Americans with Disabilities Act. But even with these accommodations, it takes a lot of courage to keep trying. She

---

[21] O,Neill, J. "Hoosier man proves climbing mountains is mind over muscles." *The Indianapolis Star*, February 26, 1995.
[22] McMorris, F. "Aspiring lawyer with dyslexia gets test access." *The Wall Street Journal*, July 18, 1997. P.B1.

very simply did not give up. Her vision of what she wants has enabled her to keep going back, even after so many obstacles. Not giving up will eventually allow her to achieve her goal. It does not sound to me as if she is looking for pity, or special entitlements not available to others whose learning disabilities require more time than average. She very simply wants to use her education to make the most of her career.

Greg Nichols has been training in bodybuilding since he was eleven years old. His dream was always to become an occupational therapist. A fall from a balcony, which broke is back, almost ended that dream. But Greg did not give up. He continued to work toward that credential because he "always wanted to help people out."[23] In 1994, he won the National Wheelchair Bodybuilding Championships, held in Palm Beach, Florida. Even faced with the worst disability a body builder could imagine, Greg did not give up. He just adjusted his sails a little.

Joanne Beckwith did not give up. A self-employed artist, she felt she needed a more secure job after being diagnosed with multiple sclerosis; so she enrolled at Loyola Law School and graduated in the top fifth of her class. You would certainly agree with me that law school is an awfully tough mountain to climb on the way to a "more secure job." But the ability to "never give up" must be what kept Joanne going. In November of 1996, she received the good news that she had passed the California Bar Exam. Her specialty is dealing with health, labor or employment law. Joanne looked forward instead of backward when she realized that she

---

[23] Lamson, S. "A wheelchair sport." *Quickie Chronicles*. July/August, 1994.

needed to make some different career choices for herself. Never giving up was the way she scaled each hurdle[24].

Franklin Delano Roosevelt spent from 1928 until his death in 1945 in public office. He was afflicted with polio in 1921. Despite his physical limitation, one of FDR's prime contributions in the 1930's was the revitalization of the spirit of the American people. In the words of his wife, Eleanor, "...Probably the thing that took most courage in his life was his meeting of polo and I never heard him complain...He just accepted it as one of those things that was given you as discipline in life. And with each victory, as everyone knows, you are stronger than you were before.[25] How lucky are we that he never gave up! In fact, FDR's disability added to his personal appeal because it made for a more poignant success story, one the American people could champion.

Abraham Lincoln said, "I will study and prepare myself and one day my chance will come." Very little greatness is ever achieved without a good amount of persistence.

The law of statistical probability says that the more you try, the more likely you are to succeed. It may take a long time, but in the meantime you have a "goal," and you can "see the winning." Your resolve never, never to give up will keep your eye on success.

Barbara Jordan did not give up-ever. She was elected in 1966 as the first Black in the Texas State Senate and in 1972 as the first Southern Black in the US Congress since

---

[24] National Multiple Sclerosis Society, 1996.
[25] Goodwin, D. **No Ordinary Time**. New York: Touchstone,1994 ,p.80.

97

Reconstruction. "But the hurdles she cleared before entering politics were just as formidable…..After graduating from law school in 1960 (where Black women, in that city, at that time, were second-class citizens)…Miss Jordan had the temerity to believe she could practice law. And she did, often representing indigent clients in disputes against the police…..It was, perhaps, Miss Jordan's own sense of humor—her basic optimism about life, her good will and her appreciation for the absurd-that helped her overcome personal obstacles. She used a wheelchair since the early 1980s and was said to have multiple sclerosis."[26] Barbara Jordan was, and always will be, my hero. She died of pneumonia in February of 1996. For those of us who have had the fortune to hear her great oratorical talents, a great voice has been silenced. And, of course you know that she had many challenges before which she would not give up. As she continued to meet political challenges, she figured out the way to get things done in Congress. She "was coming to work and I wanted to get that message across personally.[27]" Barbara Jordan faced many challenges in Congress, in addition to her declining health. She had to muster support to continue the Voting Rights Act against terrible odds. Had she not been persistent vs. antagonistic, it would have been an uphill battle. In this way, Barbara Jordan showed us that it is not enough just to be persistent; you have to be persistent in a way that will get you the support you need. In other words, you have to "never give up" in a friendly way.

---

[26] Hirsch, J. "Driving Miss Jordon." *The Wall Street Journal*, January 19, 1996.
[27] Rogers, M. (1998) **Barbara Jordan, American Hero**. New York: Bantam Books (p.113).

I have many heroes in the "never give up" category, as you can see. But last Christmas I was treated to the story of Zoe Koplowitz[28], the slowest runner in the New York Marathon. In 1996, she came in last—she came in 28,657[th]. To quote from her book, _Winning Spirit_, "Not just last, but dramatically last: 27 hours and 36 minutes after beginning on the Verrazana-Narrows Bridge at 6 a.m. on the previous morning." Zoe Koplowitz has multiple sclerosis. If you think that I felt like a slug when I finished her book, you are right! I gave up my running career when I could no longer run because it seemed like the thing to do. But not Zoe! She takes this course with two Canadian crutches, lots of friends such as the Guardian Angels to get her through rough parts of the city, and more grit than I can even imagine. Zoe Koplowitz is the spirit of Never Give Up. Picture this: In 1995, Zoe starts off in an icy rain, driven horizontally by the wind. It takes her more than an hour to get across the Verrazano bridge, normally a half-hour's journey. By the time Zoe and her companion get across the bridge, they are frozen, wet, and their hair is covered with icicles. When I read this, I felt like a worse slob because I would have given up at that point. Even I, who has surmounted major career and educational obstacles, would have given up at that point! But she has done this nine times! That takes real courage, or, in my grandfather's lingo, chutzpah! Maybe one of the passages in the book can help explain this because this has been important to me, too (though not to the extent that I am willing to survive freezing rain by choice:

> _That sense of not taking things_
> _for granted is very important to_

---

[28] Koplowitz, Zxoe (1997). **The Winning Spirit**. New York: Doubleday.

me. It is one of the gifts that MS has given me over the years, the certain, irrefutable knowledge that nothing in life is a given. Nothing is forever. It can all be snatched away from us in an instant[29].

Winston Churchill had to repeat the eighth grade three times because he could not grasp English. In October,1941, at the height of World War II, Harrow School invited him to return and speak to the young students. You can imagine how excited the students were to hear the greatest Englishman of all time address them! The following is from **The Secrets of Power Performance**, by Roger Dawson[30], a book that I highly recommend:

He stood up and looked out at the boys for a long, long time before he finally spoke. ......Finally, he gave his entire speech in just a few words, "Never give in, never, never , never, never—in nothing great or small, large or petty—never give in except to convictions of honor and god sense." Then he sat down."

I have to admit that many of my successes in life have been because I did not give up. I can remember several

[29] Ibid,p.131.
[30] Prentice Hall, 1994.

instances of being told that we were not getting the business by one buyer or another, and then finally getting it because I did not give up on that first negative response. I remember being told that no woman had ever made it and no woman ever would when I tried to break into the food brokerage business in Southern California. I proved them wrong and became salesman of the month within six months! Not giving up, though, requires a lifetime commitment. As we agreed before, motivation is not permanent, but neither is bathing! Like personal hygiene, we must continue to persist for the rest of our lives. When we are knocked down, as all of us have been, we need to get back up. I think the ability to rise from adversity and keep going is what separates many of our most admired statesmen and leaders from average people. But if you are reading this book, you are not average! You are someone who wants to take responsibility for your life. I can think of no better way than refusing to give up on a daily basis.

What do you want to do? I have a friend who wants to start a new career that requires a graduate degree in psychology. She has heart problems, a tumor, and multiple sclerosis. Her friends think she is crazy. I do not. She reminded me of a discussion I had several years ago with someone else about the rigors of a Ph.D. program. I felt that I might not be smart enough to get a Ph.D. because of memory and concentration problems that accompany multiple sclerosis for some people. But my friend said that all it takes is persistence. Never give up!

If NEVER seems like a long time, think of it as one day at a time. You can do anything for one day, such as stop smoking or stay on a diet. It shortens the never and makes it livable. I read a column in "Dear Abby" around the New Year that we could apply to these desires:

> *Just for today, I will live through this day only, and not set far-reaching goals to try to overcome all my problems at once. I know I can do something for 24 hours that would appall me if I felt I had to keep it up for a lifetime.*
>
> *Just for today I will be happy.*
>
> *Just for today I will adjust myself to what is. I will face reality.*
>
> *Just for today.....*

Just for today, I can try to walk, ride my exercise bike an extra five minutes or you can read a book about your goal, work on strengthening your body, eat a healthy diet so that you will have the strengthen to tackle tomorrow's goals.

CONCLUSION

I have enjoyed this journey with you. I hope that you have as well. My purpose was to encourage you to look at your life in a number of ways--things you can do given your disability, ways you can help others while helping yourself, ways to look at your life that will give it more quality. We all have a very short time on this earth, and you deserve to get the most out of it. I hope that you have been thinking about your life's objectives during this journey, and that you will pick one of the chapters to use as a basis for furthering your objectives with even more meaning.

You have so much to offer that only you can offer! Each and every one of us is different, with different talents and different desires. Anyone you admire has a number of things he or she does not do as well as you. You have a perspective on life that the able-bodied and emotionally well cannot appreciate and would benefit from learning- from you!

There is always so much to do when we are trying to count our blessings, use our talents, help others, work on family relationships and make other choices about our everyday lives--all at once! But I really believe that we can get more out of our life if we get the most out of every day with which we are blessed. Of course, taking this entire process one step at a time gives it a structure that adds to its attainability!

Whatever you decide, the most important thing to understand is this: *If It Is To Be, It Is Up To Me*--because it is! No one has the right to tell you what you have to do with your life; that is your responsibility and your responsibility alone. You always have choices and a chance to make more choices as you learn more about your abilities and the opportunities that are out there.

Today really is the first day of the rest of your life. I wish you love, and I wish you life. Most of all, I wish you the full realization of what you have to give and receive in return for the blessings you have been given. The blessings we each have been given.

So use your talents and use your choices. You will never have a better chance!